THE WISDOM OF
LIVED EXPERIENCE

THE WISDOM OF LIVED EXPERIENCE

Views from Psychoanalysis, Neuroscience, Philosophy, and Metaphysics

Maxine K. Anderson

KARNAC

First published in 2016 by
Karnac Books Ltd
118 Finchley Road, London NW3 5HT

British Library Cataloguing in Publication Data

A C.I.P. for this book is available from the British Library

ISBN 978 1 78220 212 7

Edited, designed and produced by The Studio Publishing Services Ltd
www.publishingservicesuk.co.uk
email: studio@publishingservicesuk.co.uk

www.karnacbooks.com

CONTENTS

PART II
VARIETIES OF COMING ALIVE

PART III
BECOMING AND BEING

ACKNOWLEDGEMENTS

Creative efforts require generosity from many sources. Here are some who have aided the emergence of this book.

Deep thanks to the following publishers for their kind permission to cite from these works: Yale University Press for permission to cite from *The Master and his Emissary: The Divided Brain and the Making of the Western World*, by Iain McGilchrist; Karnac Books for permission to cite from *The God of the Left Hemisphere: Blake, Bolte Taylor, and the Myth of Creation*, by Roderick Tweedy (Karnac, 2012); Stanford University Press for permission to cite from *Difference and Disavowal: The Trauma of Eros*, by Alan Bass (copyright 2002 by the Board of Trustees of the Leland Stanford Jr University).

A special thanks goes to Rod Tweedy, whose editorial advice and encouragement have been a compass amid uncertainty throughout the project.

I feel indebted to my long-time friends and colleagues, Mary Kay O'Neil, George Moraitis, and Jerry Jacobson, Ladson Hinton, and Elie Debbane, whose thoughtful comments about the scope of the book and style of writing have been so helpful. And to colleagues and students with whom I have studied and learned so much over the years; our often mutual collaboration has been deeply enriching and indeed inspiring. And to the best of my teachers about the inner processes of the human mind and heart, my patients, who have entrusted me to aid in their deepest explorations; I feel grateful and honoured for each of those opportunities.

Finally, inexpressible thanks to my husband Al Francisco, who has been a true partner in this effort. His prodigious reading has brought forward many references I would not have otherwise encountered. His significant technical skills have kept the manuscript organised. And his ongoing patience and encouragement, including lattes at 4.00 a.m., have nourished mind and heart throughout this whole endeavour.

ABOUT THE AUTHOR

Maxine Anderson, MD, trained in psychoanalysis in both the US and London, England. She is a training and supervising analyst for several psychoanalytic institutes in North America. She is a Fellow of the International Psychoanalytical Association and has published widely on psychoanalytic topics especially relevant to contemporary Kleinian and Bionian thought. Her most recent explorations into the nature of reality attempt to bridge the disciplines of psychoanalysis, neuroscience philosophy, and metaphysics.

FOREWORD

We live in exciting times. In just the past ten years, we have learnt so much about both human and artificial cognition, from breakthroughs in neuroscience to amazing developments in machine learning, and every year this trend seems to accelerate. While I am writing this foreword, a computer programme has convincingly beaten one of the strongest Go masters, almost twenty years after the chess champion Kasparov lost to the Deep Blue computer. An amateur Go player myself, I had not expected to see the Go champion lose to a computer in my lifetime.

It is becoming clear that a grand experiment is under way, accelerated in the past few years, in which the philosophical mind–body problem has been catapulted to centre stage in everyday life. Disruptive innovation, based on huge scientific and technological breakthroughs, is changing the landscape of our world and the way we look at our own minds. Artificial Intelligence (AI) is bringing us self-driving cars. Robots are finally getting out of laboratories and factories, and the Internet of Things (IoT) is starting to connect sensors, gadgets, and machines everywhere, creating an intelligent fabric of infrastructure for tomorrow's world, which is already appearing today.

As a result, we hardly have time even to begin to integrate all the new insights into a coherent view of who and what we are. And, in the middle of all that, how and where can we hope to find ways to let all of our new knowledge mature, ferment, and transform into new forms of wisdom? What can we carry over from the past and what is it that needs to be replaced?

Descartes asked these questions in his *Meditations*, in the turbulent days of the dawn of modern science, and our current age asks us the same questions with more urgency, given the growing imbalance of the impact that science and technology are making on the world. It is as if all of us are now thrown into a collective myth, in which we are stripped of what we thought we are, and are not yet sure of what we may become.

Many ancient myths start out with a hero-to-be leading a comfortable life, up to the point that external circumstances force him or her to move way outside his or her comfort zone. A period of great turmoil follows, after which, finally, a totally new kind of comfort is found, unimaginably different from the stale and stagnant pseudo-comfort at the start of the story. The freshness and richness of the newly discovered comfort can be seen as a discovery of a form of authentic Being that is timeless, even though the becoming is pictured as a narrative in time. The process of dis-covering is, indeed, that of an uncovering of what is most deeply human through a process of heroic battles with hardships.

Until the not-so-distant past, those myths carried an essential therapeutic value, helping us to move from more limited and limiting forms of comfort to wider and richer forms, through upheavals in between. It starts with the painful process of birth, a necessary stage in becoming fully human; it is repeated in the period of puberty, with all its doubts and uncertainties, and it replays itself for each of us, to greater or lesser extents, at many twists and turns in our lives. However, just now, when humankind collectively is facing the largest upheavals that we have ever faced, the ancient myths strike us mostly as quaint and outdated.

Yet, the same theme still operates: the challenge to start from a time-bound, limited, and relatively innocent version of comfort (paradise), through a time-bound process of forced and forceful becoming, to the possibility of uncovering a kind of timeless liberation from the doubts and anxieties that hindered progress. It is this possibility that Maxine Anderson illustrates through a fusion of her life-long clinical experience with her interest in applying the latest scientific insights, to help us rise beyond our tendency to fall back on the half-remembered, half-imagined comfort of the past.

The hallmark of addiction is turning one's gaze towards the past, in an attempt to repeat what seemed comforting then, over and over again. We see this on an individual level with any type of addiction we find around us. We see it also on a global level, with all major countries tending to succumb to the lure of twentieth-century promises of progress through reductionist science, and nineteenth-century promises of state formation that are being reworked repeatedly. What we need is a truly twenty-first century way of systems thinking, respecting both the reductionistic basis for knowledge and the way that complex systems show emergent behaviour that, as such, can never be found merely in the parts of the puzzle that is life.

To sum up, I encourage the reader to read this book more than once. At first, as an invitation to understand one's own struggle with the limits of rationality, in growing respect for awe that transcends a measuring and prematurely evaluating, reductionist mind-set. Then, as an invitation to view the struggles of others, not only individually, but also in the groups that present themselves in our society, from family to colleagues, to any organised or spontaneously appearing tribe of any kind. And, finally, as an invitation to view the way we are so far failing to provide a sustainable path for the future of our planet. On all three levels, this book offers us hope: no matter how dark the intermediate challenges are, while there is never a guarantee of redemption and liberation, there are many clear paths towards moving beyond the time-bound restrictions that we find ourselves currently believing in.

Returning to our new confrontation of the mind–body problem, in the decade of the twenty-teens that will be remembered as the breakthrough of artificial intelligence, what we need are bridge builders between the past and the future. Anderson is one of those, courageously taking the lead, paradoxically not as a leader, but as a fellow traveller.

Piet Hut
Professor of Astrophysics, and Director of the Program in
Interdisciplinary Studies Institute for Advanced Study,
Princeton, New Jersey

PREFACE

Over 2,000 years ago, in the midst of the authoritarian culture of the Roman Empire, a poem was written which invited the reader away from the trappings of power, prophecy, and superstition, so prevalent at the time, towards another perspective: one of nature based on a clear, calm view of the world as comprising the eternal ebb and flow of indivisible particles that the Greeks called "atoms". The Epicurean Roman poet Lucretius, who authored *De Rerum Natura* or *On the Nature of Things* (Smith, 2001[1969]), draws one away from adherence to dark superstitions and the dread of powerful gods and towards the value of a tranquil life based on one's own experience, as defined by the senses and the moment, while also being guided by reason and the quest for happiness. The poem encourages appreciation of the beauty of the natural world, including one's balanced passions, and gratitude for being part of nature, based on the physics of freely flowing atoms rather than the rage of the gods. The resulting gift of freedom from shame, guilt, and fear is one of the deep attractions of the point of view this poem puts forward.

These Epicurean ideas were, of course, a threat to the power-based structures of the state and, later, the Church, which might be part of the reason why the poem fell into obscurity for over 1,000 years.

However, it was rediscovered in the early 1400s by a disenfranchised Church official named Poggio Bracciolini, who might have been looking for ancient texts to counter the corrupting influences of power, intrigue, and greed he felt to be rampant in the Rome of his time. His careful preservation and distribution of this poem is felt to have encouraged the attitudes which took root in the Renaissance and beyond: art which sprang from the value of the senses and immediate experience; sciences, based on observation, as pioneered by Galileo and Newton; political thought such as that of Thomas Jefferson, who was known to have owned several copies of the poem and whose phrase "the pursuit of Happiness" penned into the Declaration of Independence, is some evidence of his being influenced by the Epicurean sentiments (Greenblatt, 2011).

The quest and journey of Poggio, movingly conveyed in Greenblatt's *The Swerve*, reminds us that we each search out "the nature of things" in our own quests for depth and meaning. In the past several years, my own search as a psychoanalyst has been for ways to understand deeper realities initially inspired by Wilfred Bion's notations about "becoming": that we cannot approach the deeper aspects of reality by intellectual and verbal means; the ever-present flow of such realities that evade the grasp of thought and conscious observation can only be approached as we can trust in our more primary modes of embodied, lived experience. Coming upon McGilchrist's *The Master and his Emissary* (2009), then, was for me like encountering Lucretius' landmark poem: this significant work considers the many aspects of cerebral laterality, emphasising the interplay as well as the distinctiveness between the wide-ranging attention and inclusiveness of the mostly unconscious right cerebral hemisphere and the more conscious, detailed, fine-tuned, language-based functions of the left.

Most significant in my quest toward becoming has been McGilchrist's and other sources' emphases on the primacy of the right hemisphere, which, while quiet, is also very sturdy. Not only does it quietly register embodied, intuitive experience, but, as illustrated by the powerful poetry of Blake and the personal experience of Bolte Taylor, its internal focus may sturdily illuminate the tyranny of the intellect. Doing so reveals the frozen constraints of insistently held positions to be the products of brutal division, rather than unassailable "truths". This capacity to look below the surface and to reveal obscured aspects of reality fosters the softening of hardened positions, which facilitates integrative acceptance. The right hemispheric functions, then, become the portals to our deepest wisdom about ourselves, and about reality.

McGilchrist, thus, inspires sojourns into other perspectives which form the basis for this book: the importance of the dialectical process in psychic awakening as well as in growth and evolution; the primacy of affect that gives rise to hallucinatory phenomena and to some forms of trauma, while also providing the energy for cognition; the importance of implicit, unrecallable memory and learning; the depth and meaning of the poetic. All of these are avenues toward "becoming and being".

This book, then, is an exploration of contemporary understanding from philosophy, neuroscience, psychoanalysis, and metaphysical studies, which seem to verify the value of the Epicurean sentiments in terms of the wisdom of lived experience. In addition, interestingly, it might portray the authoritarian culture which Lucretius felt to be the Rome of his time, to be seen in our time as the world view which the left hemispheric functions depict, that is, a narcissistic view which encourages power, greed, and self-interest—alluring attributes during the past two or more centuries in western thought.

Introduction

As suggested in the Preface, this book explores various aspects of the nature of reality and, more specifically, that of lived experience. In recent years, I have become aware that my efforts to learn from theory and from noted colleagues have often meant closing down my experiencing mind and focusing upon the intellectual and the theoretical, rather than upon the more three-dimensional lived experience with my patients and within myself. Wilfred Bion, an author whom I admire, encourages learning from one's own experience, while allowing any thoughts derived from the reading of his and others' works to become part of one's accruing understanding. Yet, this advice, which trusts the intuitive, seems to be difficult to follow. What seems to happen more, at least among students of psychoanalysis, is a close, almost scriptural study of favourite authors as if to unlock the secrets that those texts themselves might hide. Here again, idealising texts and theories as if they hold deeper wisdom than does one's own experience.

So, when I came upon Iain McGilchrist's book, *The Master and his Emissary* (2009), especially his depiction of the left and right brain interplay, and, in this instance, how the intellectual left brain so needed for language and abstract thought can obscure the softer implicit aspects of lived experience, I felt I had a companion in terms of the dilemma I had encountered in my endeavours towards deeper learning about human nature and, perhaps, about nature itself. The question that posed itself almost naturally was what are the significant elements in the process of coming alive that are essential for incorporating the intellectual and the intuitive toward the multi-dimensional qualities of lived experience?

This book, then, is a tracing of my explorations of this complex question. The sequence of the book describes the path of my own searching. I begin with McGilchrist and other sources, employing an emphasis on the intellectual, left-brain manner of looking closely at the research and honouring the texts. It is not until later in the book that I am able to turn to my own inner experience, including dreams and clinical work. It felt imperative to "do the research" first, to read what others have thought, before I could turn to my own experiences. I believe this is in accord with the scientific approach of gathering the data and gleaning others' contributions as one gains footing about one's own potential offerings. However, such can also be the path towards idealising the intellectual, which might freeze the frame that then rejects new considerations. This could be the case especially when that frame involves the valued work of mentors and others with whom one might identify.

Later in the book, I begin to set out my own explorations, including my dreams and clinical experience. The tone then changes to a more interior exploration. It is hoped that the reading of the book will aid in answering that question about the process of awakening, or coming alive. Here, then, is the travelogue of my journey.

Chapter One focuses upon the importance of the dialogic interplay which seems so vital to coming alive: first, in terms of left- and right-brain functions as noted by McGilchrist, who emphasises the co-operation between them but also their creative opposition and different views of the world. Next, the dialectic of *Aufhebung*, as noted by Hegel, which involves the creative transformation of elements as from bud to flower to fruit which seems relevant to all of biology, perhaps to all of nature. Then, psychoanalytic understandings about the birth of the subject, the birth of the "I" as noted in the works of Freud, Klein, Ogden, Civitarese, and Siegel. As well, what processes impede that developing subjectivity, what resistances to growth and differentiation are inherent in us all? Bass's work on disavowal as the response to disturbing realities is informing here.

Chapter Two deals with neuroscience, which is verifying the importance of sensory-based functions as essential for the deepening integration of the subjective self, some of that being the enhanced appreciation of the primacy of the quiet right-brain functions. There is significant focus on the recent work of Mark Solms that emphasises the primary nature of affective consciousness along with its inevitable accompaniment by intrinsic emotion. Also shared are ponderings about the myth that consciousness is a high order attainment of the cerebral cortex. Later chapters suggest that this myth might derive in part from the propaganda that left-brain functions broadcast about the primacy of cognition. An additional consideration is that this conviction might serve as a shield from the innate terror of one's poorly mediated affects.

One stunning suggestion of Solms is the tendency toward automatisation, which seems inherent in thought-based functioning: if all learning can be relegated to unconscious processing, then the need for consciousness wanes. The echoes of this tendency towards somnolence and its countermeasures are reviewed as well. The work of Friston regarding free energy and its destabilising potential offers new ways to think about intense, unmediated affect—that is, as unbound free energy. This chapter concludes with a review of the experience of Jill Bolte Taylor and her left-sided stroke as a compelling testament to the very different views of reality that left and right brain articulate.

In Part II, the focus turns to other processes of coming alive. Continuing to appreciate the primacy of affect, it highlights how innate expectations might be the roots of unconscious fantasy, the ubiquity of hallucinatory phenomena, and the creative contributions of poetic states of mind.

Chapter Three notes that evolution and foetal experience might hard-wire the anticipation of a caring environment. The suggestion here is that innate or prenatal stirrings might be considered to be the roots of unconscious fantasy. As well, the roles of implicit (the earliest and unrecallable) memory and explicit (conscious) memory are considered in terms of their significant impact upon affective, lived experience. An example of a dream of a young child is offered to illustrate several elements described in the chapter.

Chapter Four looks at how much of reality is composed of hallucinatory phenomena. That is, sensory input, such as the remembered dream, that arises from *internal* sources. It appears that we are virtually hallucinating all the time. In addition, this chapter considers aspects of psychic trauma in terms of affective overwhelm and the crucial role of negation and cortical shaping as part of necessary regulation. The fundamental nature of hallucinatory experience as a basis of lived experience, but also as primary to our identity, is considered. A personal dream is offered to illustrate some of these concepts. Here, the tone of my writing shifts from the perhaps dense considerations of others' work to the softer relating of my own experience.

Chapter Five continues this change in tone, demonstrating how poetry, as an example of the more intuitive approach to coming alive, bridges the cognitive and the contemplative, the left- and the right-brain approaches to experience. This chapter also illustrates how the metaphoric capacities of the right brain foster such depth of view. In addition, via the powerful poetry of Blake and Milton, this chapter offers the opportunity to view the poetic depiction of the tyranny of the intellect, and the measures necessary to end its rule through both recognition of that tyranny and the reintegrative potential that accompanies that recognition.

Part III attempts to consolidate aspects of coming alive that are also considered in terms of Bion's concept of becoming. Chapter Six draws together several threads of understanding thus far. It begins with a reminder that we construct reality from what we expect to see, as illustrated by the humorous experiment of the unseen gorilla on the basketball court. It continues with an illustration of how the bud-to-flower-to-fruit of Hegel's *Aufhebung* illustrates an evolving, transcending process, which can be seen in dialogue and, more generally, in the differentiating processes of living organisms. It also focuses on how the poetic state of mind can enhance and deepen self-awareness. This includes tracing the myth of the Garden of Eden as the journey of the mind from the medieval paradise of absolute truth to the more modern daring to step into the unknown with its attendant doubts amid uncertainty. This departure from the Garden of the absolute might lead to the grace of an open dialogic stance that offers receptivity, learning, and change. The resulting potential for enhanced inner space is described and illustrated with a personal vignette. A brief discussion of the neurobiological view of mindfulness is then offered, which illustrates heightened capacities for integration of affect and cognition, suggesting enhanced capacities to bear psychic pain without collapse. The latter portion of the chapter offers a brief discussion of two authors' works that reflect this open stance amid trust and faith—Wilfred Bion and David Bohm. The basic themes of being and care as also seen in the philosophy of Martin Heidegger are mentioned. In conclusion, a comparison and contrast of the various faces of reality as viewed by Bohm and Bion is offered as a touchstone to the internal dialectic between the implicit and explicit aspects of experience.

Chapter Seven traces my personal experience over the years from the intellectually based definitive thought gained in medical training to the seeking of the more open-ended learning from emotional experience. I describe my experience of how mind closing adherence to theory may be, but also how I discovered that one's attribution of authority to others might also shut down the mind. I trace my explorations of reaching beyond my discipline, including a sojourn in the virtual world to study the nature of reality. Notations of my own experience as well as those from the leader of that exploration are included. I then relate some details about an experience which seems to have fulfilled the previously not fully formulated goals of my search—an experience of a non-authoritarian group organised around learning from each others' clinical material, in a several-day workshop located in beautiful surroundings. It seemed that these circumstances fostered the open dialogic stance suggested by Bohm and the late Bion in which there may be true learning from one another's experience in a receptive, trusting atmosphere, which fosters the emergence of deeply creative contributions from nearly all members of the diverse group. Key elements for this openness seem to be mutual respect amid a non-authoritarian atmosphere. The creative emergences might have been fostered by that receptivity.

This chapter, then, emphasises once again the sense of an innate expectation of attentive care, perhaps the equivalent of non-judgemental curiosity felt in the dialogic group, and its crucial role in terms of fostering one's coming alive, that is, one's becoming. Residing in that receptive atmosphere amid trust and awe, remaining open to be moved by, and to learn from, evolving experience and genuine dialogue might be considered as approaches to being.

Chapter Eight, "Epigenetics", as a burgeoning new field, raises the question of the impact of immediate lived experience upon genetic expression in all animals studied. Compelling evidence is offered as to how immediately genetic expression at a cellular level can be affected. In some cases, dramatic change seems to occur within minutes. Amid heated debate within the field about these new findings, it might be that, as yet, we do not know how to think about these data in terms of what is really occurring.

However, if the immediacy of experience really does have an impact that can last into future generations, we might need to be open to new ways of thinking about its significance. If the learnings of this book have any validity, it will be important to remain open to as yet unglimpsed aspects of reality, which might lead to new realms of understanding about the power, as well as the wisdom, of lived experience.

PART I

GATHERING PERSPECTIVES ON
LIVED EXPERIENCE

Introduction to Part I

Part I examines some of the concepts about coming alive, the birth of the experiencing mind.

Chapter One reviews philosophical (McGilchrist, Hegel) and psychoanalytic (Freud, Klein, Winnicott, Civitarese, Ogden, Bass, Siegel) views about the birth of subjectivity, the birth of the experiencing "I".

Chapter Two considers neuropsychiatric views (McGilchrist, Feinberg, Solms, Friston, Siegel, Bolte Taylor) that are verifying the importance of sensory-based functions as essential for the deepening integration of the subjective self. It also reviews the paradigm shift in the neuroscientific work of Solms, Damasio, Panksepp, and others, which emphasises the primacy of consciousness inevitably accompanied by intrinsic emotion. This shift prompts one to ponder why, for over a century, there was a general agreement amid psychology and psychoanalysis that consciousness itself required cortical deciphering. The assumption has been that wisdom of experience lay with the cortex. Later chapters try to address this myth of wisdom residing only in cognition, which might be due to the propaganda that left-brain functions broadcast.

Dialectic origins

W e each face a paradox: our adult selves want to grow, but we hate to be disturbed. These differing basic tendencies, encountered by most living things, it seems, have apparently triggered a response which embraces both poles of the paradox. That is, openness to the new alternating with a closed-ness to maintain stability and continuity. In our human experience we have an ongoing to and fro that allows growth and differentiation within the limits of what is bearable. We are open to the new until anxiety and fear of discontinuity intervene. And then, once closed, the continuing wish in health to grow eventually overrides the anxiety of change leading to an opening of the system again. When harmonious, this to and fro may be considered as part of the ongoing process of coming alive, or what Wilfred Bion notes as "becoming".

He reminds us that, while we rely much on "knowing about" in order to learn about the world and ourselves, it is only through immersing ourselves in lived experience, what he calls at some points being, and at other points becoming, that we can approximate the complex multi-faceted experience of the wider, deeper reality which Bion denotes as "O".[1]

Something very much like this underlies/drives the process of physiological system change. It is an interdependent process of "becoming" we LIVE our healing

Bion (1970) and others, such as McGilchrist (2009), suggest that emphasis on intellectual endeavours often brings imbalance, for our tools of knowing can hamper the wider wisdom that emerges from living in the moment, a wisdom that allows us deeper access to reality.

Becoming involves the often courageous registrations of encounters with emotional truths and other painful experiences, such as suffering the guilt which attends one's becoming responsible, facing the loss and mourning the wastage when confronting one's entrenchments and destructive behaviours, and facing the unknown, unshielded by the illusions of certainty or seeming possessions of the truth. All of these facings and livings involve disturbances to our everyday selves. Bion stresses that becoming involves those indescribable, multi-dimensional experiences that can only be *lived* in ongoing ways (Bion, 1970, p. 28).

body

In this regard, I am reminded of my experience of being with a patient, or, indeed, with a close friend or family member in which there is deep resonant interchange, much of which is out of awareness, and then of my trying to write up the hour or take verbal note of the deep discussion. My efforts at this notation often feel like sorting through a heap of dried leaves. The multi-dimensional experience cannot be adequately captured by words or retrospective thought. Only in resumption of the contact, as in the next analytic hour or the renewed conversation, can the fullness of the *lived* experience be resumed.

In trying to think further about lived experience, I found it useful to look to new, unsaturated views and several authors especially caught my attention, as they were each speaking about a similar theme: of nature as an active process in which reality is created via a continual dialectic process of differentiation. I will try to outline these viewpoints as they relate to the underlying processes of becoming.

?

McGilchrist: the dialogue between the hemispheres

Iain McGilchrist's *The Master and His Emissary* (2009) richly depicts the effects of the harmonious to and fro of the right and left cerebral hemispheric functions in the evolution and elevation of man's emotional, spiritual, and intellectual development. While this work is intriguing for several reasons, I try here to focus on its relationship to lived experience. His work also directed me to the writings of the German philosopher Hegel, and especially his concept of *Aufhebung*. In addition, I also found the recent work of Alan Bass and the more current work of Giuseppe Civitarese, as well as the reflections of Tom Ogden on the dialectics of Freud, Klein, and Winnicott, and Dan Siegel's work on the integrating function of emotion very informing about what vitalises lived experience. I shall try to summarise my understandings, that is, my own dialectical process, in considering these works.

McGilchrist might be at the forefront of the emerging literature of interest to psychoanalysts on the significance of cerebral lateralisation. Drawing upon many careful clinical observations of normal functioning, as well as the disruptions of bilateral harmony through stroke or disease, he richly demonstrates the complexity of the ever-flowing interchange between right- and left-brain functions. However, he also raises the question of whether it is more appropriate at this point in our understanding to consider these opposing, and yet complementary, functions as metaphors about the different ways of being which comprise human experience. In my own studies for this book, encountering various neuroscientific viewpoints about laterality, while also appreciating the danger of proclaiming an absolute reality, I have felt it best to generally refer to right- and left-brain functions and ways of being. This stand, I feel, respects the complexity involved in the complementarity while also noting the clear distinctions that each hemisphere brings to lived experience.

Briefly, the right hemisphere involves the intuitive, implicit, mostly unconscious, sensory-based experience, in the moment, which remains open, receptive, and wide-ranging. It comes online in development before the left hemisphere and remains orientated to the input from the body but also to otherness in terms of the world beyond the bodily self. This otherness includes care from and of others.

In addition, it is attentive to the many levels of affective experience which emanate from within the individual as well as from the outside world and it seems to be instrumental in the unconscious origins of thought as noted in unconscious gestural and affective expressions (McGilchrist, 2009, pp. 41–44). These functions, which offer orientation to oneself and the world from earliest infancy, play vital roles in the individual's lived experience, probably comprising the "ongoingness of being", concept basic to Winnicott (1960).

However, the left hemisphere is also important in this regard. Its functions, which become active from about eighteen to twenty-four months of age, are those which link to the realm of conscious control of oneself and environment as it relates to the world. These include focused attention, fine motor co-ordination, development of language, manipulation of objects—in short, those qualities that allow for the exploration and the conquering of nature and her secrets. With regard to the interplay between the two hemispheres, the left seems to have the capacity to render explicit, that is, to bring to consciousness, the implicit unconscious messages offered by the right hemisphere. It brings clarification in symbol and language to that which emerges from the unconscious, but, in doing so, it separates the clarified and the symbolised from the dynamic in-the-moment experience. It will be up to the vast associational networks of the right hemisphere that foster metaphoric function to animate the symbol that the left brain has established. An example of this interplay is a sensitive, accurate interpretation: the labelling function of the interpretation helps to establish and strengthen the symbol (left hemispheric function) while the experience of the receiver feeling deeply seen and understood provides enlivenment (right hemispheric function). Finally, it will be the right brain that reintegrates the newly animated symbol to become part of the unconscious roots for the next intuitive processes (McGilchrist, Chapter 2, p. 5).

Relating to the different views about self and the world, McGilchrist and others (Bolte Taylor, 2008a) mention that each hemisphere, perhaps because of its neural circuitry and the information it processes, seems to have developed a specific attitude: that of the right (which processes input simultaneously) as open, compassionate, non-judgemental, and patient, reminiscent of a sturdy compassionate parent, probably linked with the primary tasks of assessing and responding to the environment in a patient, receptive, reliable fashion. The attitude of the left hemisphere appears to be very different: processing input in more sequential fashion, rather like a child searching for mastery and caught up with its own productions, this attitude tends toward focused exploration, domination, and power, relating to anything outside of its own efforts as something to master, to manipulate, or to dismiss. In addition, as McGilchrist and Jill BolteTaylor (2008a, p. 53) emphasise, the left treats its efforts and inventions as non-living specimens. Just as its approach to the world is mechanical and manipulative, it cannot bring the spark of life to its efforts. The left clarifies what emerges from the unconscious realms monitored by the right. Bringing vitality, what is commonly thought of as heart, remains a function of the right hemisphere. Further, it has also been observed that the left hemisphere appears contemptuous of anything it has not created, including the softer, less articulated integrative functions of the right. This is probably due to the intensity of its declarations, which come with language and the ever-present so-called evidence of its products (things, ideas, would-be certainties), which we are likely to find so alluring because these evidences and intensities are so familiar and so front and centre in our everyday experience.

In health, then, McGilchrist presents evidence that the right brain senses and presents implicit messages that the left brain then clarifies and symbolises. However, as mentioned, it is up to the right to bring vitality to what has been symbolised, which occurs as that message is enfolded back to become the root of the next intuition. This enfolding back into the implicit is the most vulnerable step in this dialectic because the left brain resists giving up the products of its so-called invention (thoughts). Giving up for the left requires faith that the overall product (ideas that nourish the next intuition towards ongoing growth of the organism) will be worth the surrender of the prize. The right hemisphere, relating to integration, has the faith, but the left, which is more orientated to control than surrender, may override that faith, out of the grasping certainty that it is foolish to not hold tightly to what one has invented.

My main damage [handwritten marginal note]

Hegel: transformations from bud to flower to fruit (Aufhebung)

McGilchrist (2009, pp. 203–207) suggests that the co-ordinated effort between the hemispheres is an elegant example of the concept of *Aufhebung*, a concept introduced in the early 1800s by the German philosopher, Hegel. This concept provides a guide for a universal process of evolution and transformation involving the simultaneous alteration and preservation of vital aspects of what has gone before. Hegel suggests the model of the flower bud transformed into the blossom and then into the fruit as suggestive of the model of alteration and preservation in the carrying forward of vital biological processes.

A number of papers by Jon Mills (1996, 2000, 2002) make Hegel's work quite accessible and psychoanalytically relevant. My comments come mostly from Mill's papers.

Hegel wrote several volumes on the growth of the spirit, his term, which approximates our modern term, ego. One of the most influential aspects of this work that has come down over two centuries is his concept of a dialectic form, *Aufhebung*, that apparently applies throughout nature. It is often paraphrased as involving "thesis, antithesis, synthesis", a triad of terms which might be misleading in that one may surmise that there is a complete cancellation of thesis and antithesis by synthesis. This assumption would neglect the subtle but essential preservation and elevation of aspects of each phase by the process. What is truly important in *Aufhebung* is the sense of creative elaboration and growth, rather than the more reflexive annihilation of the opposition, the latter being a pattern that might seem painfully familiar in certain political, philosophical, and, indeed, psychoanalytic discussions where there is no wish to learn from the other or to change one's position.

Hegel's attribution to the growth of spirit or ego towards Truth involves this process of ongoing experience of thesis (the new idea or experience of truth), which, when submitted to the opposition of doubt, or antithesis (bifurcation and division), is mediated so as to allow it, after sufficient examination, to be viewed as an aspect of truth worth noting, rather than as a frozen absolute or universal which was probably the ego's first response to its otherness. The final stage of this cycle is synthesis, when the examined foreign object, seen now to be potentially enriching rather than threatening, is welcomed as part of the self. During this and subsequent cycles, the self is learning about itself and the world, advancing towards truth, in Hegel's terms.

A brief reference to the familiar theatre of our own experience might add clarity to this concept. To my quiescent self, any disturbance, such as a new idea, initially feels like a threat that I reflexively treat as an alien, not-me element in order to examine it and also to maintain my repose. This means that I externalise this seeming threat (via a left brain function), making it a devitalised foreign body (a "threatening" idea) against which I erect a clear, rigid boundary. This now externalised disturbance may remain as a frozen, unchanging foreign body (an ongoing threatening Other) unless I (or someone) can employ the left brain function of examination and clarification and come to realise that this foreign-seeming element can become an informing piece of new information (an idea that can offer new insights), which I can then reincorporate via right brain functions. My realisation and reclamation revitalises that former threat, as it becomes part of my newly enriched self.

There are several important elements in this dialectical cycle: disturbing difference triggers tension, rigidity, and disavowal, which give rise to a distancing from, and scrutiny of, this now deanimated specimen. Examination and clarification (left-brain functions) can only be done from afar. The right-brain function is necessary for the vitalising reincorporation and enrichment by the now digested disturbance. This might be the most vulnerable aspect of this process, for, as mentioned, it is difficult for the left brain to surrender its hard-won prize (the examined specimen); it wishes to grasp and to hold on to what it feels it has created, oblivious to the wider task of reintegration for the growth of the entire self. Another very important aspect of *Aufhebung* involves the birth of subjectivity ("I-ness"), which occurs as the self can come to see itself not just as reactive to the perceived threat, but as an agent, an *observer*, of the foreign object.

For Hegel, this continually enriching process is self-generated and self-revealing. For clarity, the negation at work here is seen in the alienating not-me functions of projection, deanimation, and examination, all left-brain functions. The process of examination, however, especially while it freezes and, thus, renders the alien into a de-animated specimen, also alters the experience of the disturbance by allowing it to become just one aspect of ongoing experience rather than a *tsunami* of disturbance. In addition, the mediation fosters the burgeoning awareness of the self as agent, as an observer of this process, and this self-awareness ushers in the birth of subjectivity.

Ogden: the birth of the "I" in psychoanalysis

Psychoanalysis is replete with examples of the dialectical processes exemplified by Hegel and McGilchrist. Tom Ogden has written several significant articles reviewing Freudian, Kleinian, and Winnicottian perspectives on the birth of subjectivity (1992a, 1992b). His descriptions vividly suggest that coming alive, that is, the birth of the subject, requires the space created by, and within, a vitalising dialectic.

Regarding Freud's contributions to this coming alive, Ogden (1992a) mentions how the conscious and the unconscious realms represent two different ways of being, each defined in terms of its opposition to the other. He makes the repeated point that the unconscious–conscious dialectic is in constant oscillation, giving the illusion of a unity of experience, as does the interplay of id, ego, and superego in their constant dialectic dialogue. His succinct descriptions deserve quotation:

> In Freud's schema, neither consciousness nor (dynamic) unconsciousness holds a privileged position in relation to the other: the two systems are "complementary" (Freud, 1940[a], p. 159) to one another, thus constituting a single, but divided discourse . . . (Ogden, 1992a, p. 518).

Freud's final model of the mind recalls three aspects of the self: the id as the original erupting force which cannot be directly known but whose force is ever impactful; the ego, which is that aspect of this force which becomes the conscious "I"; and the superego, as an emergence from interaction of the primary force and the external environment which aims to guide, but often torments, the self. In this model, the subject, that sense of "who I am" comprises the ongoing dialectic between these three aspects which creates "a stereoscopic illusion of unity of experience" (Ogden, 1992a, p. 520).

Regarding the Hegelian emphases on negation and transformation, Ogden reminds us that Freud's paper "Negation" (1925h) illustrates the dialectic at work, where a repressed idea or image can become conscious if it is negated, that is, not accepted (e.g., "I am not concerned about X"). He also emphasises that the fullness of experience, from a psychoanalytic view, necessitates the to and fro between presence and absence, affirmation and negation. The power of transference exemplifies this as an emergence of experience from the consciously forgotten past into the immediacy of the present. Both past and present are affirmed and negated; both past and present are present and absent.

Turning to Melanie Klein's dialectics regarding the coming alive of the subject, Ogden (1992b) suggests that at least three of her concepts involve relevant dialectical interplay: the oscillation between paranoid–schizoid and depressive positions, that is, between separation and integration; the to and fro between the splitting and the integration of the subject, and her concept of projective identification. As poles of an ongoing dialectic, Klein's positions offer a distinctive way of conceptualising modes of experience, differing in emphasis from the developmental models, which suggest a more linear sequence. Klein's paranoid–schizoid and depressive positions decribe two oscillating modes of experience, which are in constant dialogue. The paranoid–schizoid way of being is based on sensory experience and immediacy, enacting impulse, having no sense of past or future, and, indeed, having no real sense of the I-ness of the subject. The depressive position, the other pole of that dialogue, is that in which there is a sense of I as subject and observer, or agent. Klein suggests this is the position in which one can appreciate the whole and the complexity in oneself and in others. Due in part to the survival of sturdy compassionate objects, the violence of the splitting mechanisms recedes, tolerance of tension and frustration has become more available, and the capacity for continuity and ongoing-ness provides the space needed for greater depth of experience and meaning to evolve.

Besides offering a rich discussion of the creative dialectics of the paranoid–schizoid and the depressive positions, Ogden (1998) also has written compellingly about a third mode of experience, the autistic–contiguous, which he links with the other two modes to form a three-way dialectical interchange. He suggests that the autistic–contiguous position comprises sensory-based experience, that is, the senses and rhythms that form the earliest shapes of experience, prior to the emergence of a primordial sense of self and other.[2]

The dialectic between these positions, the individual oscillating between the paranoid–schizoid, depressive, and autistic–contiguous positions in everyday life, brings to the fore the panoply of maturity, primitivity, and subjectivity. The oscillating dialogue between integration and closure and the necessary splitting or breaking up of that closure allows for new combinations of unconscious internal objects and ego integration, which can only lead to a more creative and complex interchange between inner and outer worlds of experience.

A summary of the impact of the splitting mechanisms, from Ogden's view, on the internal landscape and the relation of splitting to narcissistic functioning might include the following: splitting is involved in the defensive regulation of pain when there is resistance to fully feeling the grief of loss which would involve mourning. It also attempts to master or regulate, rather than to tolerate, pain. The melancholic who cannot bear to face the pain of real object loss, to face and to truly accept it, withdraws to a narcissistic level of relatedness and identification with the lost object. Instead of the pain of mourning and acceptance of loss, the melancholic experiences depletion, often sadism and revenge, but retains a fantasy of control and ongoing entanglement with the object by way of identifying with that object, by becoming it in fantasy. Unconscious internal objects that are shaped by splitting mechanisms, such as the melancholic entanglement with the lost object, cannot be involved with learning from experience. Splitting, instead, does the opposite; it keeps the ego in fragments, amid an atmosphere of pressure and potential violence.

Addressing the violence often incurred in splitting, Hinshelwood (2008) suggests that what is involved is a violent shattering of experience, usually following what feels like a violent assault or confrontation. Where repression involves a substitution for a repressed affect, splitting leads to an absence, an annihilation of the unbearable affect or content. Close attention to the process will probably reveal that the mind that utilised splitting itself felt violently attacked.[3]

However, for balance, the creative aspects of splitting, its contribution to coming alive, are also important to consider: the splitting processes in their disintegrative function also give rise to new possible recombinations, new experience. Splitting may, in *Aufhebung*, contribute to the automatic creation of the necessary distance needed to view as alien that which is new or disturbing, and, thus, it might be an automatic mechanism developed in evolution to tell friend from foe. From this view, splitting, in its unconscious automaticity, assures the organism an efficient process (thinking fast rather than thinking slow) while, significantly, aiding the development of discernment and possibly the sense of self-consciousness.

Ogden (1992b) also addresses Klein's concept of projective identification and its interpenetrating nature as the *inter*personal component of the dialectic of integration and deintegration of the subject, but his attention turns mainly to Bion's modification of Klein's concept in terms of the container–contained concept. He emphasises the mutual interaction within the dyad as "the creation of subjectivity through the dialectic interpenetration of subjectivities . . . [where] projector and 'recipient' (infant and mother) enter into a relationship of simultaneous at-one-ment and separateness" (p. 618). Each member of the dyad, then, is giving shape to the other.

Ogden feels that the work of Donald Winnicott advances the psychoanalytic conception of the birth of the subject beyond the dialectics established by Freud and Klein (1992b, pp. 619–620). He notes that one of Winnicott's great contributions regarding the lived experience of the subject is its simultaneous existence in the space between the inner and outer world, the "transitional space" half created by phantasy, half by encounters with external reality (Winnicott, 1953). He elaborates four forms of Winnicott's dialectic involving coming alive, all denoting the evolving relationship of the mother and baby. One of these forms, "primary maternal preoccupation", which is described as the mother's capacity for nearly full identification with her infant while at the same time retaining her separateness, is a very early form of the to and fro between oneness and twoness. In this phase, the baby attains the sense of "going on being" which precedes the sense of an individual self, but which lays a secure basis for continuity (Ogden, 1992b, p. 620).

The second Winnicottian concept in terms of the subject coming alive is the "'I–me' dialectic of the mirroring relationship" (Ogden, 1992b, p. 621). Here, Ogden sensitively suggests that in the mother's role of mirroring her baby back to him, she reflects back slightly differently from what she sees in her baby. This crucial difference allows the baby to feel seen as an "other", as "experiencing the difference between self-as-subject and self-as-object" (Ogden, 1992b, p. 621). He suggests that a crucial internal space is created in this dialogue of slight difference.

A third Winnicottian dialectic, involving the transitional object, is the to and fro between the object being created and the object being discovered. The unchallenged existence of the paradox between "created" or "discovered" coincides with the unchallenged presence of the mother as available, but able to play a quiet background role. This stage then allows the baby to experience his mother both as an external object and also as his own creation, as her being there for his needs alone; it precedes "the capacity to be alone" which occurs when the child can come alive as his own subject without needing to "create" the mother for his sense of continuity (pp. 621–622).

The fourth Winnicottian dialectic cited by Ogden involves this capacity to be alone. Winnicott refers to this phase as the baby's "creative destruction of the object" (Ogden, 1992b, pp. 622–624). This concept has been difficult for many to discern. Ogden's view is that there is a difference between relating to mother as an object, that is, as a repository for the baby's needs, wishes, and projections, as dictated by his being unable to see beyond the sphere of himself as the centre of the world, and relating to the mother who can be seen as welcoming the baby, insistent demands and all, without retaliation or rancour. While neither Ogden nor Winnicott say this clearly, I believe the implication is that this phase sees the shift away from the violence of the splitting processes via mother's patient tolerant presence in the face of that violence. When the baby can see beyond the jagged world of his insistent demands, beyond the pressure of his own affective upwellings and his own omnipotence, he can glimpse a patient, sturdy, compassionate mothering presence who has not been damaged by, or become retaliatory to, his violence. This survival and emergence from violence, again, due to the good enough compassionate persistence of the mother and the baby's tolerance of his/her own temperamental upsets and capacity for a changing view, signals a shift in the baby's own capacity for subjectivity. The pressures of splitting give way to the quieter potential space for hope, amid time and reflection upon the other as a full human being. This capacity to reflect upon the damage of one's own violence brings the capacity for guilt into being. Hope, patience, time, and space become possible, enhanced by the mother's capacity to embrace all these elements of her baby with reasonable patience and care. The creative destruction of the object then can be considered as the dialectic to and fro, which allows containment of the baby's violent experience when he is in the grip of the splitting processes.

A summary of Ogden's discussion of the dialectical creation of the subject, of the experience of "I-ness" in terms of Freud, Klein, and Winnicott, can be offered in the following:

> Emanating from a continuous process of dialectical negation ... the subject is always *becoming* through a process of the creative negation of itself ... The constitution of the subject in the space between mother and infant is mediated by such psychological–interpersonal events as projective identification, primary maternal preoccupation, the mirroring relationship, relatedness to transitional objects, and the experiences of object usage ... (Ogden, 1992b, p. 624)

All of these dialectical processes echo the basic processes of *Aufhebung* (Ogden, 1992b, p. 624).

Civitarese: the vitalising function of maternal reverie

While Hegel poses a self-revealing system toward growth of the mind, Giuseppe Civitarese posits the mother's attention and reverie as part of this crucial animating role. As he updates Donald Meltzer's writings on the aesthetic conflict to focus on the earliest engagements of the merged mother–infant dyad, Civitarese echoes the principle of *Aufhebung* as he invokes the most primary somatic rhythms, attunements, and slight discrepancies as essential in laying the groundwork for the baby's emergence from the undifferentiated reality, while also maintaining the vitalising link with it.

Echoing Hegel, Civitarese says, "The aesthetic conflict is thus an expression of the very dialectic of reality, that is . . . (the oscillating) logic of identity and difference . . . of *Aufhebung* . . . through which the individual emerges from undifferentiation" (2013, p. 151).

He speaks of these differentiating processes as "necessary fictions, or lies in terms of the undifferentiated realities" (Civitarese, 2013, p. 112). In addition, he comments on how Bion and Hegel consider *not possible* reality as primarily the quietude of the inorganic state, and the birth of the individual involves differentiation away from that inorganic reality. This ongoing differentiation takes work and involves clashes with the undifferentiated real that are felt via emotions. True thoughts, from this vertex, go toward de-differentiation, entropy, and death, while false thoughts, dissonances, and those elements that animate, "gain the vital gap of subjectivation" (Civitarese, 2013, pp. 112–113). Civitarese suggests that there needs to be a balance between the de-differentiating pull towards and differentiation from the inanimate real for the individual to live in the world but also to maintain his individuality and thought. These balancing, integrating functions are probably primarily right-brain mediated, as this region is linked with vitality, integration, and depth of view.

Civitarese continues to outline the vitalising function of the mother's attentive ministrations, as "the device for constructing symbols . . . necessary for facing up to the real" (2013, p. 112). The mother's reverie is her way of tempering the undifferentiated aspects of reality to the needs of her child, thus making the real tolerable for her infant.

He mentions how Bion's concept of the alpha function mediates and transforms: how the mother's rhythms transpose sensory experience into meaning, how her attunement matches, but also augments, the infant's emotion in ways which aid the baby's coming alive to encounter rather than to avoid his/her emotions (Civitarese, 2013, p. 150).

All of these animating, integrating functions would probably be primarily right-brain functions, as they are so closely related to bodily cues and rhythms, but also to the associational networks of the right brain which foster the interconnections needed for metaphoric function.

Bass: differentiation as disturbance, disavowal as response

Having explored some of the dialectics relevant to the birth of the subject in Freud, Klein, Winnicott, and Civitarese, all of whom consider aspects of the dialectic between mother and baby in terms of the increasing sense of separateness which includes internalisation of otherness, we turn to an author whose view of the dialectical process adds another dimension of depth and complexity. Alan Bass (2000) offers a compelling argument that the recognition of differentiation inherently includes the potential trauma about loss, a trauma which, at some point, triggers defensive disavowal, a situation which creates two realities—that which welcomes differentiation and growth and that which opposes it in attempts for stasis and control.

While Hegel writes about process triggered by the urge towards life as disturbing the quiescence, Alan Bass writes about similar processive patterns from the perspective of difference and differentiation as disturbance. Taking Loewald's preference of nature as differentiating process, rather than nature as the assembly of created objectified entities, Bass parallels Hegel, McGilchrist, and other authors we are citing in terms of reality having a basic emphasis of ongoing processive development.

Bass's significant studies on concreteness and fetishism lay the groundwork for his understanding of a normative oscillation between a dynamic reality where differences can be appreciated and growth may occur and the static, frozen reality where time and space collapse and no sense of difference can exist.

From his close study of concreteness, triggered by how impervious the concrete patient is to content-orientated observation or interpretation (1997, 2000), Bass concludes that the process of disavowal of difference which occurs unconsciously from early in life is one that actually precedes and displaces repression as perhaps the major organiser of psychic life.[4] These concerns relate to the process known as fetishism, which might be a universal defence when the need for stasis and continuity prevail.

Fetishism relates to the terror of the recognition of difference, and the need to repudiate that recognition by substituting concrete, opposing, firmly bounded fantasies of relieving presence and tormenting absence. It was not until late in his career that Freud (1927e, 1940a) acknowledged the likely primacy of disavowal and splitting of the ego over repression in terms of the basic organisation of mental life and psychic reality. Bass, and others, have carried this line of Freud's thought forward. With homage to Loewald (Bass, 2000), he suggests that we all experience the unconscious registration of a dynamic differentiating reality in terms of a caring environment, which provides sustenance to the needy self. An unconscious registration of satisfaction would exemplify this universal state. Such a basic need-satisfying environment not only provides sustenance and growth, it also raises tension around the absence of those supplies which, at a certain point for all of us, might become too much to bear.

Bass suggests that disavowal is employed in order to erase from memory this disturbing reality about potential loss. Disavowal, which leads to concreteness, unconsciously registers the nurturing environment and, thus, acknowledges potential differentiation, but then it erases from consciousness the awareness of that fluid process involving the humanising links with the nurturing environment (gratitude for nurture). It imposes, instead, the frozen field of intensely held, dehumanised, concrete fantasies experienced as absolute, unquestionable reality (convictions experienced as absolute knowing and, thus, absolute control). These concrete fantasies derive from what Freud and others identified as perceptual identity ("what I see is what is real"), that pre object-orientated reversion to the immediate sensory experience as "all there is". This reversion to perception as reality, then, invokes the same hallucinatory processes that mediate the remembered dream. That is, the products of perception are experienced as all of reality. Freud spoke of the eradication of memory in this process as "negative hallucination" (Freud, 1917d). Bion would later refer to this as "breaking the links", collapsing the space for the appreciation of difference of thought and plunging the individual into the flatland experience of frozen scenes and unchanging absolutes based entirely on sensory intensity.[5]

The narcissistic need to control reality in order to maintain an equilibrium, which involves obliterating the awareness of ongoing differentiation, then, means that one enters a hallucinatory world and experiences it as all of reality. This aspect of reality comprises rigidly bounded, polarised, concrete fantasies. The defensively concrete individual experiences like-mindedness as soothing ("agreeing with my position is 'understanding' me"), but difference is experienced as agitating or hostile ("your non-agreement is your 'being mean' to me"). Confrontation with difference then might be experienced as a play for power, or even as seriously destabilising for the individual in a defensively concrete position.

A clinical vignette might aid in conveying the feel for the intensity, even desperation, of the concrete experience, as well as the disorientation which could occur when differences in reality are encountered.

Years ago, a patient of mine, caught in a concrete state of mind, was struggling with my non-alignment regarding multiple requests for changes of the frame, which he described as "reasonable requests". Initially, I had granted these requests, but each time I did he had a dream of a mad old woman, which we both came to understand was me, the analyst, agreeing with the request rather than holding the frame; at first, this learning from the dreams brought my patient relief that a deeper issue might be revealed and understood, but soon thereafter the "reasonable requests" returned and the memory of the lessons from the dreams was lost. Quoting from the paper in which I reported this case,

> One day he was especially caught up with my "not getting it," again meaning that if only I knew how hurt he felt and how rigid he saw me to be, then I would change my position about the request. During this hour I felt that I could see the situation more clearly: what I saw was an . . . impoverished-feeling infant-self locked into an entrenched position such that no degree of parental understanding could touch or move . . . him. I suggested to him that he felt so deeply entrenched . . . [that none] of my so-called understanding [could] be of help to him, and that the only way he felt we could find accord was for me to change my mind. He felt (to his surprise) that he was seen clearly in terms of the entrenched stance but [he] was also *disoriented, unsure if my seeing his entrenchment was my tricking him, seeing him clearly, or changing my stance.*

As we investigated this disorientation, I suggested that when he felt so clearly seen, in fact the . . . embattled part felt there could be no difference in our points of view because that part could not envision difference that was not threatening. (Anderson, 1999, p. 509, emphasis added to underscore the confusion felt when my patient felt clearly seen)

The consequences of this defensive reversion to the concrete can be dramatic in terms of lived experience. Within such a firmly bounded, claustrophobic experience, there is no sense of an abiding presence or gratitude, or the capacity for reflective thought. Rather, one feels an overriding sense of pressure and dread with no sense of escape or emergence. The cost, then, to defensively reduce the tension accompanying differentiation might be high. We sacrifice our humanising links with uncertainty for the inhuman stasis. The splitting we have employed to get rid of tension-raising difference also, in Bion's terms, might shatter our capacities to contemplate the different possibilities embedded in reflective thought. We exist, instead, in a debris field made up of mutilated bits of mental functions etched by grievance, suspicion, and dread.

When difference disturbs us deeply, we might draw upon the narcissistic illusions of self-sufficiency and control via freezing the frame, over-valuation and idealisation of parts of the self, or, indeed, things within one's possession. We might resort to entrenchment as one form of fetishistic response or we might select an over-valued or idealised object, convinced of our safety and strength in its presence and our vulnerability or impotence in its absence. These behaviours, or objects, could include sexual fetishes, good luck charms, entrenched positions, or over-valued fantasies, ideas, or theories.

Anything that interrupts the awareness of an ongoing, fluid differentiating reality by means of a riveting focus upon a static, over-valued thing or position may be considered to be serving fetishistic purposes.

Thinking about this in our everyday lives, we all are familiar with slipping into the illusion that we "know what is best . . .", or "what the other guy is thinking . . .", or ". . . my idea is threatened if it is not the best idea in the room". We each have a narcissistic base of imagined self-sufficiency and omnipotence, which Bass notes as a "defensive counter-surface" that comprises intensely felt concrete fantasies intended as protection against the unknown and the uncontrollable aspects of reality. However, as we grow and have more space and tolerance for various ideas, we may be able to allow the right-brain functioning of tolerance and integration to mediate the left-brain insistence and illusion of possessing the best and only possible idea.

From McGilchrist and Hegel's views, we oscillate between right- and left-brain clarification and right-brain reintrojection. We each, then, can oscillate between differentiation and de-differentiation, between many views amid uncertainty and the narcissistic insistence of knowing the "truth" or having the answer.

A few added thoughts about the hallucinatory aspects of concrete fantasies might be useful: as mentioned, Bass suggests, and the clinical vignette offered may illustrate, that the intensely felt concrete fantasies ("your not agreeing with my reasonable stance is your being so mean to me") act as a counter-surface, or rigid skin, that serves as would-be protection against the unknown and uncontrollable. Yet, a signature feature of concreteness is that it bypasses the perspective and dimensionality which *memory* (in the vignette, losing touch with the shared learning from the dreams) provides in terms of assessing reality. Concreteness relies entirely instead on the products of immediate perception, that is, from sensory stimuli arising from internal sources (his distress at my non-compliance was equated with my being mean to him). Looking closely, all narcissistic phenomena geared toward defensive self-sufficiency comprise such fantasies, often held as convictions (my patient's entrenched certainty about my meanness) and, thus, are actually hallucinatory in nature. Yet, in everyday life as well as when one is steeped in an entrenched position, there is a need for these hallucinatory constructions to bolster a sense of boundary and identity, of "who one is and what one knows". So, again, it is interesting to consider that our boundaries of self, needed for everyday life, largely comprise hallucinatory phenomena—"necessary fictions", as Civitarese might say—for our well-being.

Bass advocates a therapeutic approach that is not so much geared towards addressing the content of the concrete fantasies and insistences as towards addressing their defensive function. That is, why is it so important to the individual to maintain a sense of certainty and stasis in the face of difference? As evidenced in the vignette, the differentiating function of the neutrality of the therapeutic setting (holding the frame rather than agreeing to change the time), which triggers narcissistic frustrations and resistances, brings this conflict right into the consultation room. Addressing the fear of loss and instability (how painful it is when I do not comply), bringing to awareness the process of the oscillating to and fro (the embattled part not being able to envision difference that is not threatening), and our inevitable embeddedness (my compliance at times prior to understanding the dreams) in this process aids in the wider view of reality and its complexities. Such an approach, of course, also helps the therapist to keep from falling into a fetishistic trap of his own, which might be his insistence upon his "correct view" of the situation. A major part of the therapeutic tack Bass advises involves focusing away from the closed system of certainties and objects, and emphasising more the pains and dreads of openness, of the proceeding into uncertainty which we all face, amid our human best efforts.

A couple of companion thoughts which might be difficult to contemplate at this point: the unconscious primary awareness of need and integration with another (in the vignette, the patient's fleeting relief that the lessons from the dreams might point to a deeper issue) is an aspect of secondary (differentiating) process, while the primary process hallucinatory phenomena (his distress at my non-compliance experienced as my being mean to him) which construct our narcissistic boundaries are conscious. Unconscious secondary process, and conscious primary process. The awareness of primary disavowal and fetishism, as Bass has delineated, alters traditional views of psychic makeup, which may be clarified in Solms' (2013) work.

The overriding message of Bass, Hegel, and others, is that the psyche comprises a process of oscillation between differentiation, towards change and growth, and de-differentiation, assuring continuity via stasis.

Siegel: mind, brain, relations as three aspects of one reality

Dan Siegel's interpersonal neurobiology (IPNB), as exemplified in his book *The Developing Mind* (2012), is resonant with many of the previous authors mentioned. IPNB suggests that "mind, brain, and relationships are not three separate elements, . . . (but are rather) 'three aspects of one reality'—that is, energy and information flow" (p. 7). Here, "information" is described as "swirls of energy that have

symbolic meaning". These three elements—brain, mind, and relationships—influence one another recursively to give rise to emergent, self-
organising processes that tend towards integration.

Siegel stresses the fundamental role of emotion as both the vehicle
carrying forward the flow of information and as a way of organising
various aspects of neural development: as we recognise and regulate
our emotions, we regulate ourselves.

> Emotion, as a series of integrating processes in the mind, links all
> layers of functioning. In fact, the study of emotion itself is essentially
> the study of emotion regulation. Although emotion can be defined as
> a subjective experience involving neurobiological, experiential, and
> behavioural components, it is, in fact, the essence of mind. . . . Siegel,
> 2012, p. 306)

As part of the integrative process, Siegel describes the development of mind as illustrating complexity theory, in that the emergent
processes undergo both differentiation and integration. Differentiation allows specialisation, such as of the various peripheral senses,
the subcortical and cortical brain functions, the implicit and explicit
memory systems, the multiple levels of emotion, the right- and left-
hemispheric functions. These differentiated elements are then linked
into harmonically resonating states of mind or ways of being when
all goes well. The most promising harmonics occur when the most
benevolent attachment patterns with primary carers have occurred.
Siegel emphasises how these attunements from a sturdy, sensitive,
compassionate mind foster linkages in the growing mind that tend
towards both mental and emotional continuity (familiarity) and flexi-
bility (openness to the new). However, as mentioned earlier, in terms
of enlivening metaphor such a sturdy sensitive presence also estab-
lishes a sense of "feeling felt", an affirmation of one's subjectivity,
which helps to establish new dimensions of experience. Siegel's
emphasis upon the crucial role of the interpenetration of minds in all
aspects of mind–brain growth underscores the view of secure attachment, attention, and compassion as vital building blocks in emotional
development and, thus, self-regulation as well as other enriching
consequences of human development.

> Early in life, the patterns of interpersonal communication we have
> with attachment figures directly influence the growth of the brain

structures that mediate self-regulation. . . . Emotional communication . . . is the fundamental manner in which one mind connects with another. (Siegel, 2012, p. 306).

Vital for discussions of lived experience are Siegel's integrative thoughts about emotion and modes of repair of the disturbing disharmonies that could develop. He suggests that the attunement between therapist and patient allows for resonance of right-brained and left-brained functioning in both parties. The right-to-right would be a feeling of being felt or affirmed, and, thus, recognised, bringing a sense of a recognising other into the patient's experience. The left-brain language description of these affirmations leads to the "name it to tame it" distancing which language allows, freeing the individual from being caught in the sweep of the unnamed emotion while fostering verbal thought about those states. These resonances, both non-verbal attunement and shared language, Siegel suggests, foster integrative growth and a sense of an accompanying mind, first externally in the therapist, later becoming internalised as part of one's own integrated and integrating self (Siegel, 2012, pp. 333–335).

CHAPTER TWO

Neuroscience emphases on lived experience

Contemporary neuroscience brings some interesting perspectives to the exploration of lived experience.

McGilchrist (2009) gives a lengthy discussion of detailed aspects of left- and right-hemispheric functioning. While he mentions many times how important the harmonious functioning of both hemispheres is for development, his focus is on the distinctions between the hemispheres rather than their similarities or the overlap of function. His many examples focus on the two ways of viewing the world: the up-close meticulous examination of the left-brain functions and the more contextual and wider view offered by the right. He also repeatedly suggests that the depth of experience fostered by the right hemispheric functions has been eclipsed by the vividness of the front and centre focus on language, precision, and mastery, in which the left excels. He suggests repeatedly that we are fooled by the allure of the left in its promises of clarity, and have overlooked for centuries the quiet depth and wisdom offered by the right hemisphere. This wisdom, carried by non-verbal communication, is echoed by several authors (Divino & Moore, 2010; Pally, 1998; Schore, 2011).

Schore, Feinberg, and Salas and Turnbull
on the primacy of the right hemisphere

Allan Schore, whose monumental work *Affect Regulation and the Origin of the Self* (1994) is a compendium about the impact of affect in the evolution of the psyche, boldly supports the implicit functions of the right hemisphere as playing the dominant role in human experience (Schore, 2011).

> Despite the designation of the verbal left hemisphere as "dominant" due to its capacities for explicitly processing language functions, it is the emotion-processing right hemisphere and its implicit homeostatic-survival and communication functions that are truly dominant in human existence. (pp. 76–77)

Schore emphasises the role of the right brain in processing emotion and the impact of primary relationships such as the intimate interactions between the mother and baby, which are registered in the right orbitofrontal cortex. His work, which spans two decades, underscores the central role of these early experiences in forming the sense of a seen, felt self, so reliant on the sensitive, responsive caring environment.

He also mentions several aspects of right-brain mediated implicit or non-conscious phenomena: projective identification, which is that feeling that something has been lodged in one by someone else, often with powerful impact, is described by Schore as right-to-right hemisphere communication which bypasses the conscious regard offered by explicit memory and attention. Transference, where the past comes forward to be experienced as in the here and now, completely bypassing conscious awareness, also exemplifies this implicit level of experience. As well, Schore emphasises that the role of enactments and intuitions in everyday life, as well as in clinical work, are primarily registered in the unconscious right brain. This valuable review of the impact of implicit experience (2011) suggests, as does Bass, that dissociation, the cleavage of the implicit, rather than repression, as Freud had held, is far more dominant in shaping psychic development and functioning than had been appreciated.

Todd Feinberg (2010) offers further neurological evidence of the importance of the right frontal cortical regions as playing a crucial role in the establishment of boundaries of the self. He states that "right frontal damage creates both a disequilibrium in ego boundaries as well as a breakdown of the observing ego, the ability to take an outside perspective on oneself" (p. 133). I read Feinberg as strongly suggesting that the loss of this cohesion and boundaries might coincide with the sense of the loss of a caring presence which gives cohesion and the sense of "who I am" to the very young child. The significance of the right orbitofrontal cortex and the mother to child communication, so emphasised by Schore (1994, 2011), which is registered by this region, seems to be verified.

Salas and Turnbull (2010) offer confirmation and fine-tuning to Feinberg's conclusions. Citing some of the neuropsychological rehabilitation literature, they suggest that the matter of mature (modulating) or immature (evacuative) defences seems to depend on the capacity to tolerate negative arousal (rage, psychic pain). Patients with right frontal injuries seem especially unable to bear such painful arousal and, thus, might revert to those defences, which promote immediate discharge of that pain.

They also confirm, and even extend, the listing of right brain functions, noting in a collation of various studies that the right frontal cortex plays a role of regulation of skills having to do with judgement, decision making, and reasoning under uncertainty, while the posterior right cortex has the role of assembling subjective emotional experience relating to the body (p. 178).

These data would seem to confirm the suggestions of McGilchrist of the right hemisphere's function regulating integrative evaluation, embracing uncertainty and paradox, while also registering and cohering the variety of bodily experience in the moment, as well as discerning the experiences of self and others. These quiet but essential functions are all very important in the experience of vitality and its richness.

Solms: the right hemisphere and whole object relatedness

Several authors express various viewpoints about right hemispheric function, but the addition of a psychoanalytic view of these issues is very informing. Mark Solms, working as both a neuroscientist and a psychoanalyst, brings a depth of psychoanalytic understanding that reaches below the neurologic findings to offer some clarifications about the asymmetries between left and right brain function. Using clinical data from lesion studies, he states that the differences of function between left and right hemispheres is found primarily in the associational areas of each hemisphere. That is, the occipito–temporo–parietal junction in the posterior cortex of each side of the brain (Kaplan-Solms & Solms, 2000, Chapters Seven and Eight).

Initially, Solms reviews the basic neuroscientific understanding of the functions of these regions: the posterior cortical region associates and integrates sensory input from the external world with memories of previous experience. Specifically, the left associational area primarily receives and processes auditory and verbal input into speech and language, while the right is specialised for visual and spatial orientation and cognition. These differences lead to significant specialised functions in each hemisphere. The left focuses primarily on the elaboration of language, which aids symbolic thought, self-reflection, and the inner speech that become the basis of self-guidance (superego functioning). The right posterior cortex, receiving visual rather than auditory input, is more orientated to space, the mapping of both external space and external objects, which is accompanied also by the fostering of inner mental space. Lesions in these areas illustrate the functions each of these associational areas play in subjective experience.

From significant clinical data on lesion studies in these two regions, these authors suggest that the patient with a left associational cortical lesion loses essential linking capacities that serve to form words into coherent ideas which serve symbolisation and abstraction. Without these capacities, this patient feels as if he is in another world: fragments of thought "just happen" to him. He feels shorn of the equipment to recover coherence of skills or knowledge. Quite simply, he feels he has lost his capacity for coherent thought (Kaplan-Solms & Solms, 2000, Chapter Seven). While this can be felt as a great loss, lesions in the right associational area can be even more devastating.

It seems that the right perisylvian (associational cortex) lesions disturb deeper levels of organisation than the lesions to the left associational cortex. Typically, the patient with such a lesion has been described as consisting of deep denial of the deficit, neglect or the ignoring of left-handed space, and often disgust and even hatred towards the impaired parts of the body, which can, in extreme situations, lead to suicidal behaviour. While several theories have been put forward about the neural underpinnings of these findings, these authors, bringing astute psychoanalytic observations to this situation, suggest, compellingly, that the underlying denial, neglect, and hatred relate to the collapse of mental space and the reversion to narcissistic functioning.

The right associational cortex processes visual input relating to the appreciation of, and orientation to, external space. This includes the sense of other persons as existing in space separate from oneself. Kaplan-Solms and Solms suggest that, psychoanalytically, this orientation is considered as whole object relatedness. That is, the appreciation of the other's unique qualities. Developmentally, this is considered to be a step forward from relating to others narcissistically, that is, as pertaining to one's needs. When the capacity to appreciate and relate to space collapses, as in a right posterior cortical lesion, there is a simultaneous collapse of the subjective sense of internal space. One is plunged back from a spacious appreciation of otherness into the narcissistic position of feeling endangered and unable to bear the tensions that abound, including the overwhelming emotions about loss. Sudden regression to the narcissistic state of mind is usually experienced from within as a violent shock to the self, as it feels collapsed (the collapse of mental space) amid a debris field of mutilated parts of the self tormented by hatred and humiliation (Bion, 1957).

In this collapsed state, there is no ability to mourn because the self feels too shattered to even glimpse, let alone to face, the devastating loss. The abject hatred, then, and disgust for the damaged limb in these patients reflect both the raw sense of internal mutilation and humiliation which the narcissistically mortified patient is experiencing, and the rather primitive attempt to distance oneself from that offending limb ("my brother's arm"). Observing films of these patients' attempts to disavow their disabilities is heart-wrenching because the sensitive observer can perceive the painful edge of humiliation that the patient is guarding against as the neurological attendants ask directly about the disabled limb.

This kind of collapse, which characterises right posterior cortical damage, demonstrates the role that this region plays in health in terms of the sense of both the appreciation of external space and internal mental space. The capacity for mental space fosters patience, compassion, and a sense of harmony with the external and internal worlds—

qualities that go beyond the sense of one's boundaries and singularity, qualities that go beyond narcissism. When this capacity to appreciate space collapses, there is an internal collapse as well into a spaceless, pressured, and claustrophobic mental state in which the self might feel stuck. The lack of space prevents the capacity to observe oneself, which is needed to come to grips with the loss and to mourn. As mentioned, individuals with left associational cortical lesions have considerable physical loss and attendant depression, but having the sense of inner space intact (right cortex unimpaired) they can more readily mourn their losses (Solms &Turnbull, 2002, p. 271). While patients with right-sided lesions can make some use of the patience and compassion offered by the therapist, this capacity seems to be readily lost at the end of the therapeutic hour, perhaps signalling the fragility of that capacity due to the degree of damage incurred. The correlation of the capacity to appreciate external space with the subjective experience of internal space is intriguing. The Kaplan-Solms and Solms' (2000, Chapter Eight) discussion brings this dimension to the fore. Their summary description illustrates the fruitful union of neuroscientific and psychoanalytic views.

> We think that the right perisylvian convexity is a crucial component of the *neuroanatomical substrate of whole-object representation,* and therefore a *neurophysiological vehicle for whole-object cathexes* and the capacity for mature *object love.* The destruction of the vehicle of whole-object representation, caused by right perisylvian damage, therefore results in a loss of the ability to bind our fundamentally ambivalent attitude towards the real object world, with all its frustrations and privations, and therefore to an inability to relate to objects in a mature and balanced way. (pp. 197–198, original emphasis)

As a leading figure in the field of neuropsychoanalysis, Mark Solms has been working for decades to correlate the neurological underpinnings with psychoanalytic understandings (Solms, 1997). His work has led to significant debate, cross-fertilisation, and dissention. To my mind, he has led the way to a significant reworking of perspectives, which might bridge many of the gaps that have existed between these two fields over the past century. We now turn to that key paper of 2013, which makes a compelling case for the primacy of affects.

Solms: affect precedes and empowers all cognition and the cerebral cortex is unconscious while the brainstem is both conscious and intentional: paradigm shift

The traditional view, apparent in nearly all of Freud's writings, and much of the neuroscientific literature as well, has been that the cerebral cortex is crucial in the manifestation of consciousness, that the waves of arousal or potential impulse arising from the reticular activating system of the brainstem have been thought to gain consciousness via processing by the somatosensory cortical systems. Consciousness and ego were thought to be located in the cortex while the more primitive, impulse-carrying id was felt to be located within the deeper, subcortical structures. This view went virtually unchallenged for decades in the psychoanalytic and neural science literature.

Solms (2013) opens his paper entitled "The Conscious Id" reminding the reader that there are two kinds of consciousness: affective consciousness, which arises from the brainstem and registers the homeostasis from the interior of the body, and cognitive consciousness, which registers external bodily states via sensory and motor registrations in the sensorimotor areas of the cortex. He stresses repeatedly that all consciousness, whether registering internal or external stimuli, originates in the brainstem, in the extended reticular activating system (ERTAS). Again, that cortical functioning, which does register the exterior world and the body, depends on the brainstem activation.

He also cites several significant authors' work, which state that the seat of consciousness is experienced in the form of affect ("feeling like something") which emerges out of the upper brainstem. In addition, he stresses that specific basic emotions are inherent in these arousals, giving them the status of instincts, the best known being those of Panksepp (2013), who cites seven BASIC EMOTIONS (stated in small capitals to distinguish them from more everyday connotations): SEEKING, LUST, FEAR, RAGE, CARE, GRIEF, PLAY. These emotional circuits are found throughout the mammals investigated and seem to have specific biochemical sources. Solms emphasises that these circuits play homeostatic functions in biology, rather like feedback loops: the greater the emotion the more homeostasis needed to reduce that urge. The "feeling like something" is a measure of how the organism is doing with regard to internal homeostasis, intense affects being deviations from the basic quiescent state of well-being. Affect is, then, a type of reading about the inner balance or homeostasis, which can be considered as the "conscious presence" or the subject of perception, which derives from the deep structures of the brainstem. Affect gives rise to conscious experience, Solms says.

He elaborates on this paradigm shift as he states that this "subject of perception" (the "I" who perceives), which originates as affective states (initially "awakenings" and later as a more focused "I feel this way") arising from the brainstem, requires the cortical representations in order to attain the picture of what is being perceived. For every perception, and, later, every thought, there must be a subject and an object bound together in the task, the subject deriving from interior sources and the object from the external cortically registered representations. Further, Solms stresses that while all of the perceptual functions of the cortex are unconscious and derive from learning and, thus, involve memory, these cortical functions or perceptions can become conscious only when attention is paid to them, attention, of course, deriving from brainstem radiations regarding alertness which enter into feedback loops with the thalamus and the parietal lobes (O'Conner, et al., 2002; Weston & Gabbard, 2002).

What the cortex contributes, Solms stresses, is basically representational memory space, which stabilises the objects of perception, turning waves of affective consciousness into objects, that is, images, and subsequently words, which can then be used for thought. The cortex, then, is vital for giving voice, picture, and potential thought to the sensory input about oneself, including one's body, as well as gaining input from the external senses about the world.

Solms makes clear that the emotions intrinsic to the brainstem also colour the experience of core being: "*what* I feel". He suggests that basically this affective consciousness is reading and expressing the internal homeostatic well-being of the individual. It sends its readings as waves toward the cortex that in turn solidifies the affects into mental objects, which can then be thought about. The forms of memory in the cerebral cortex give representations to these waves of affects, and these representations can be sturdy enough to become objects of thought. While the representations themselves are unconscious, as is all cortical functioning,

> when consciousness is *extended* onto them (by attention), they (the
> representations) are transformed into something both conscious *and*

stable, something that can be *thought* in working memory. . . . The activation by brainstem consciousness-generating mechanisms of cortical
representations thus transforms consciousness from affects into
objects. (p. 13, original emphases)

In overview, Solms states that affective consciousness precedes
and is necessary for cognitive awareness to occur. This is a statement
that overturns a century of thinking otherwise, but it is astoundingly
close to Hegel's 200-year-old dialectical formulations in which attention examines the extruded disturbance and, through comparing it
with memory traces, comes to mediate its otherness to allow for
reintrojection and enrichment. Reaching across two centuries, Hegel
would agree with Solms. The activation by brainstem consciousness-
generating mechanisms (attention) thus transforms consciousness
from affects (disturbing feelings) into objects (representations of these
disturbances which can be thought about and enrich the self). However, attention is vital for this transformation and derives from brainstem as well as cortical sources.

Regarding the capacity to think *about* one's internal or external
experience, Solms suggests three levels of representation and abstraction: the first is the affective level of the self as subject (awakening),
the second is the representational level of self as object (aware of oneself), and the third level is the capacity to separate oneself as an object
from other objects (I see myself relating to others). This third level,
involving words and, thus, the capacity "to think about", fosters
abstract thought and, hence, self-reflection. He emphasises the importance of words and language in this function of abstraction and the
capacity for reflective thought, relevant to keep in mind regarding the
power of the left hemispheric (language) functions: "This abstract
level of re-representation enables the subject of consciousness to tran-
scend its concrete 'presence' and thus *to separate itself as an object from
other objects*" (p. 16, original emphasis). Such abstractions foster the
capacity of self-reflection.

The cerebral cortex, then, is currently considered to be entirely
unconscious in its function, serving to sculpt, to inhibit, and to transform the affective upwelling into images, words, and thoughts. The
frontal cortex also oversees the sequencing of this upwelling over time
("first this and then that . . . if this, then that"). Such sequencing intro-
duces the elements of time and space into cognitive processing and

mental time and space foster the growing capacity for self-reflection ("observing myself doing something"). But Solms also reminds us that we can be fooled by our own self-reflection:

> Because the ego stabilizes the consciousness generated in the id by transforming a portion of affect into conscious perception—mental solids (and into consciousness *about* perceptions—verbal representations)—we ordinarily *think of our selves* as being conscious . . . But this obscures the fact that we simply *are* conscious, and our conscious thinking . . . is *constantly accompanied by affect.* This constant "presence" of feeling is the background *subject* of all cognition without which consciousness of perception and cognition *could not exist* . . . The primary subject of consciousness is literally invisible, so we first have to translate it into perceptual–verbal imagery before we can "declare" its existence. (Solms, 2013, p. 16, original emphases)

I believe he is saying that affective consciousness precedes, but must find representation in order to be visible even to itself; that the emergence of wakefulness precedes all cognition but that we must utilise attention as part of affective consciousness in order to access our cortically based cognitive capacities (representations) so that we can become aware of even the existence of our being awake.

We can then read this position as affirming the primary nature of affect (affective consciousness) as the engine to power the cognitive processes, but affect also needs the representations of cognition in order to gain recognition of itself. This is very close to the position of McGilchrist and Hegel. Noting the title of McGilchrist's book, the right hemisphere is the very quiet Master (affect) and the left hemisphere is the noisy Emissary (cognition) who carries out the will of the Master by giving him voice and representation, but that it might be easy to lose sight of who is Master and who is Emissary because the (noisy) products of cognition offer themselves as evidence of being primary, and, thus, as being the Master ("we think of ourselves as being conscious"), while the true Master remains imperceptible ("we are conscious") until it has been given voice and representation by the Emissary.

Solms also deduces that when hallucinatory wish-fulfilling fantasies, which are, by definition, conscious (hallucinatory experiences are conscious), are embedded in the system unconscious, it then makes sense to conclude that the system unconscious is actually derived from experiences that were initially conscious, but were then repressed. It follows that "An innate system pre-conscious precedes the development of the system unconscious in mental maturation" (2013, p. 17). This is additional evidence of consciousness being primary, which resonates with McGilchrist's notion of the right hemisphere preceding the left hemisphere in development and also with Bass's notation of the registration of a primary (conscious) differentiating reality prior to the need to disavow it, due to the pain of loss. Thus, Solms agrees with Bass and McGilchrist: all postulate that conscious experience and registration precede the development of the system unconscious.

However, the deepest insight, Solms maintains, is that Freud's notion of two types of mental energy are verified: free energy (affective consciousness), which is conscious, and bound energy (cognitive consciousness), which aims to reduce the potential chaos which free energy engenders (Freud, 1915e, p. 188, reprinted in Solms, 2013, p. 18). Much of the paper is devoted to the discussion of the ego's effort to bind the free energy of affect, which, of course, is done by transforming it into representations, ultimately into thought with the aid of words and language. From this energy perspective, which suggests that the overall aim is to reduce the elements of disturbance, to make things more predictable, Solms suggests that the intention of the ego is to make predictions based on learning, in order to reduce surprise. The implication here, he suggests, is that the overall goal of the ego would be to learn from experience and, thus, to make such accurate predictions about the environment and the future as to allow automatisation of mental functioning. If we could relegate all ego functioning to the associative cortices as we do the functions of riding a bicycle, conscious experience would become unnecessary. This perspective, of course, bypasses the attractions of creative thought and action and appreciation of the beauty of the world. As well, the power of transference manifestations, that is, unconscious expectations that future conscious experience will replicate the past, make such automatisation highly unlikely. Unconscious fantasy can be thought about in several ways—as an inborn expectation (Bion's preconception), as an explanation or organising narrative about one's sensory experience, and as an inference about the future based on the past (transference). In all these ways, while unconscious fantasy does help to bind the free energy of raw affective upwellings, it goes counter to automatisation, and more or less assures us of a dynamic tension between "the brain . . . [as] an information-processing object . . . [and] also [grounding] an intentional subject" (Solms, 2013, p. 18).

Thus, Solms offers the hopeful prediction that the cognitive neuroscience will be open to include these inputs from affective neuroscience, including the role of unconscious fantasy, to become a more balanced mental science. Here is a psychoanalyst's wish for reunification of the affective/emotional with the cognitive, the right hemispheric functions with those of the left, the latter of which has dominated neuroscience for nearly a century.

Here are echoes of the voices of McGilchrist and Hegel about the recognition of lived experience.

Friston: unconscious inference counters destabilising surprise

Computational neuroscience is offering some ways to think about the brain, the mind, and affect, which might aid our understandings about lived experience. Beginning with basic principles, Karl Friston and others (Carhart-Harris & Friston, 2010; Friston, 2010, 2014), following Helmholtz in the 1860s and Freud, a few decades later, mention that all self-organising (biologic) systems must counter the physical law of thermodynamics that states that all matter tends toward decay and disorganisation (entropy). Living systems build towards continuity and growth, rather then entropic decay. Friston (2014) says they do so by securing a boundary that separates the self from the outside world while maintaining the continuity of that inner, growing self. However, this protective boundary must also be porous enough to allow nourishing contact with the outer world, a contact that includes the capacity to continuously update expectations and, thus, perceptions about its sensory experience of that world.

For the mathematically inclined, this demarcating boundary is known as a Markov blanket, which suggests that a blanket of probabilities surrounds and separates inside from outside, self from non-self. In the brain, this demarcation that aids self-organisation involves expectations based on probabilities: "that I will spend more of my time in this state, and less time in that one". The more familiar state then becomes the one anticipated, based on probabilities reinforced or updated by accruing experience (Friston, 2014). These expectations are equivalent to unconscious fantasies or inferences about the future based on past experience that is constantly being updated by current experience. We see this tendency towards inference in transference, because we expect in the future what we have experienced in the past. It is interesting, perhaps, to see how powerfully and subtly this phenomenon influences our perception and experience of our inner and our outer worlds. Such updating of expectations or fantasies, vital to the harmony needed for growth, then, maintains confidence about perceptions that involve the best explanations available for one's sensory experience. That is, such updating minimises the disturbing dissonance between expectations and actual sensory experience.

Such inferred explanations, which organise sensory input via a labelling process, then, protect against destabilising surprise. A good example of such is Solms' reminder that the raw, affective upwellings require registration and representation (labelling for perception to even occur) that then bind the raw affect and lead towards increasing differentiation of psychic experience. The recurrent messages, then, between raw affect and its binding by higher cortical processes, serve to shape ongoing anticipation of, and fantasy about, the next wave of affect. Thus, a continuous feedback loop, which exemplifies the binding process, suppresses entropic free energy, protecting the psyche from the disorganisation that can occur in the face of the sweep of raw, disturbing affect. Another example of a fairly common experience might be helpful: "an outrageous idea, once thought about, makes better sense"; outrage (disturbance or surprise) is bound by higher order consciousness ("once thought about"), which reduces the entropic pull so that the disturbance is mediated by sensible thought ("makes better sense").

How is this computational view of neuroscience helpful to us as psychoanalytic clinicians? In my view, it could be of help in several ways. It gives a model for understanding tension-ridden states of mind in which thought is obliterated and the mind seems to collapse. When the concretely entrenched patient encounters the wider reality that exposes his/her view as only one of several possibilities rather then the "truth", the potential for deep humiliation is significant. Here, the degree of discrepancy between the rigidly held certainty and that of the wider view might release a great deal of free energy: the individual's certainty collapses in the face of the entropic surprise, and the individual might feel a mortifying degree of humiliation. Having this model available could then aid the clinician's appreciation of the degree of psychic pain (free energy) and, thus, also the degree of defensiveness that the concrete patient might muster. Bass reminds us that the therapeutic stance toward such rigid concreteness might best be to focus on the fear of the wider view, such as "what makes it so difficult to consider that there might be other ways to view your absolute certainty about X?" This question would focus attention on the fear of exposure and humiliation, giving the patient and therapist a clearer idea about how annihilating that discrepancy might feel and, thus, how rigidly it might be defended against.

We might also appreciate, as noted in previous chapters, how potent affects, such as hate, greed, and envy may impose their intensities as unquestionable realities, collapsing the individual's ego's capacity for discernment: greed "must have"; hatred and envy "cannot bear and so must destroy". These unmodulated affects degrade potential spacious thought into pressured states of mind.

It seems as if we are driven to minimise free energy to maintain the interior as a harmonious, nurturing place. This means that we minimise uncertainty, and maximise our beliefs (our best approximations from ongoing updates) about the causes of our sensory experience. Here, we can see why doubt can be dreaded. It threatens to undermine confidence and to allow free energy to seep into the system. When one feels a threat to the needed harmony, one then encounters distress. This can be experienced as destabilising free energy, which might dissolve not only inner harmony but, indeed, one's functioning mind. The unmet insistence on affirmation in its jarring surprise, might, then, be experienced as deliberate cruelty. The unaffirming therapist, here, may better appreciate the fears of entropic collapse and, thus, perhaps address these significant dreads. That would have been a benefit in the vignette I cited about not granting the reasonable requests after learning from my patient's dreams. If I had understood this view of the entropic pull of my non-affirmation, I might have been able to address that dread and conviction more directly and, thus, more smoothly, have aided my patient's and my own exit from the near impasse.

As well, this model reinforces the essential value of unconscious fantasy and inborn preconceptions as part of the bulwark that protects the living being from succumbing to the sweep of de-differentiation. Entropy sets in when, for some reason, there is either too much surprise or too little active unconscious fantasy and binding of the free energy at hand.

This inferential model highlights another perspective on the power of reverie: the mother providing the organising function of labelling and mediating raw sensory experience, at first a maternal provision which then is gradually taken over by one's own cortical processes, one's own self-regulating ego functions. Without such a labelling and, thus, binding function available, the vulnerable self would be lost to the annihilating forces of raw affect and sensation or trapped in certain frozen disordered states of expectation as attempts to forestall that powerful entropic pull. Dissociation would be one such category, which is considered in the next chapter.

One further illustration of the power of inference resides in our consideration of the placebo effect. Until recently, the power of the "sugar pill" to bring relief and even physical healing has been puzzling. However, significant research (Ariely, 2008) demonstrates how expectations potentiate therapeutic effects: the Vitamin C pill described as an expensive medication is more effective than the "cheaper pill", which also is Vitamin C. The saline injection described as a potent drug has that effect as well for the patient, whose expectations based on hope and trust are active agents in therapeutic outcome. Growing appreciation of the power of inference and expectation sheds light on the significant effect of the previously mysterious placebo effect.

Bolte Taylor: a personal experience of left-hemispheric stroke

The vivid accounts of Jill Bolte Taylor, a neuroanatomist who, in 1996, suffered a massive left-hemispheric stroke, illustrate several aspects of Solms and McGilchrist's positions relating her experience in great detail. She offers unique perspectives from the inner experience of such trauma and recovery.

At the age of thirty-seven, Bolte Taylor, in apparently vigorous health, suffered a spontaneous rupture of an aneurysm in her left cerebral hemisphere, a stroke which, over four hours, caused her to lose the capacities to walk, talk, read, and write, and also access to the memory bank of herself and history. She vividly describes the loss and the arduous work that required years of steadfast relearning for recovery of its function. This isolation of her right-brain function allowed her to witness first hand its function once it had been released by the recession of the previously dominant left-brain function. She could also witness the quality of left-brain function, its sharp judgemental character, obsessive attention to detail and "chatter", as she calls it, as its function gradually returned. It is evident that she has become a right-brain advocate, which may place her perspective among the poets, but we might also consider her account a vivid illustration of the neuroscientific works cited above.

Her experience of the released right hemisphere led to her description about how the right hemisphere registers movement and images and that information "in the form of energy, streams in simultaneously through all our sensory systems and then it explodes into this enormous collage of what this present moment looks like" (Bolte Taylor, 2008b).

This account echoes McGilchrist's mention of wide-ranging sensory experience as the registrations of the right hemisphere. In addition, the explosion into this collage of the present moment could be an illustration of the presentations of Solms' affective consciousness in terms of right-brain sensory-based experience. In her account, energy (affective upwelling) is the coin of this realm.

Of the left hemisphere, she writes that it operates linearly and, with detailed attention, it sorts and categorises, as if to organise our memories in order to make predictions about the future (Solm's and Friston's "not to be surprised"). As it thinks in words and language ". . . that ongoing brain chatter . . . manifests my (individual) identity . . . I become a single, a solid, separate from the whole" (Bolte Taylor, 2008a, p. 142).

Bolte Taylor suggests how the left hemisphere comes to dominate the right, by focus on detail and the division and categorisation of sensory experience. In addition, the implication that such categorisation and detail creates the sense of the past and the future is an interesting emergence from left hemispheric functioning.

She speaks about how the stroke damaged the left hemisphere language centre in such a way that the inhibition that it had imposed on the right hemisphere was lifted, resulting in her capacity to view clearly the two ways of being represented by the two hemispheres.

The two halves of my brain don't just perceive and think in different ways at a neurological level, but they demonstrate very different values based upon the types of information they perceive, and thus exhibit very different personalities (Bolte Taylor, 2008a, p. 133).

[The left brain] is a perfectionist . . . [it] thrives in its constant contemplation and calculation . . . and runs 'loops of thought patterns' . . . that feel harshly judgmental, [and often] counter-productive or out of control. (p. 32)

She could look back and see the judgemental quality of her left brain as dominant:

. . . I found that the portion of my character that was stubborn, arrogant, sarcastic, and/or jealous resided within the ego centre of that wounded left brain (Bolte Taylor, 2008a, p. 145).

Via my left brain language center's ability to say, "I am," I become an independent entity separate from the eternal flow. As such, I become a single, a solid, separate from the whole. (p 142).

The stroke then relieved her conscious self of the dominant left-brain tendencies; she could step beyond the separating and categorising influences of her left hemisphere and "step right":

My stroke of insight is that at the core of my right hemisphere consciousness is a character that is directly connected to my feeling of deep inner peace. It is completely committed to the expression of peace, love, joy, and compassion in the world (Bolte Taylor, 2008a, p. 133)

These descriptions suggest several things. The distinctive character of each hemisphere is evident, and Bolte Taylor's inner experience of each character is compelling. Also intriguing is the suggestion that the information received and how it is processed gives rise to a specific attitude, a quality referred to by McGilchrist. For instance, the left brain focuses on detail, division, exactitude and we seem to experience that configuration as "driven and impatient", while the right brain is more wide reaching, never exact, and ever receptive, which we probably call "patient and without judgement". These modes of information processing seem to form the textures of our varying attitudes. Solms, and Panksepp, still might suggest that these attitudes are highly influenced, or, indeed, the manifestations of intrinsic affects, such as joy for right hemisphere and perhaps rage and anger for the left. Schore (2011) would probably feel that these attitudes reflect the nature of the intimate early relatedness with carers.

In addition, the sense of individuality sectored off by the "I am" of the left hemisphere is of interest. The right brain appreciates waves of energy and outwardly directed attention, while the left brain perceives modules of interconnected systems, clarified by detail and sequential thought. We can easily think of the right hemisphere with its soft edges, its sensory-based focus on the body and on the intuitive as being much softer voiced than the left, which commands our attention via language and linear thought.[6]

Another interesting consequence of the categorising function of the left hemisphere is the creation of a sense of time. Whereas the right hemisphere might consider all experience to be part of the ever-present now, the left hemispheric functions featuring cognition seems to utilise memory to delineate the past, and anticipation (Bion might say desire) to predict a future. The present moment might be that portion of time that cognition cannot pin down, but lived experience seems to inhabit.

Admittedly, Bolte Taylor has become a right brain advocate, but still the relative contributions of each hemisphere are stated rather boldly.

It then becomes even easier to envision Solms' contention about the cortical shaping or management of affective consciousness, as each hemisphere shapes and modifies those upwellings in a distinctive manner: the left by way of detail, division, and control via language and abstraction, the right by way of sensory experience in the here and now. Without the two hemispheres with their distinctive cognitive styles, affective consciousness would remain invisible, as it needs the sensory and symbolic components for registration. But without the brainstem upwellings, Solms stresses, there would be no energy for, and no triggering of, the cortical effects at all; in fact, he contends, without that energy there would be no life.

An added contribution of Jill Bolte Taylor is her prominently stated transpersonal experience that she felt clearly was made possible with the quelling of the dominant left hemisphere. This emphasis on the view beyond the individual gives voice to the realm of the poets and beyond in our final considerations of becoming.

A further issue which is very probably important in this case is the intimate care offered by Jill's mother: at any stage of life, close attentive empathic care is found to be very important in healing and growth. It is probable that this combination of right- and left-hemispheric care fostered the repair and reconstruction that Jill undertook. Jill's mother's patient, sturdy, and, at times, disciplined presence probably aided in Jill's being open to her debility and to learn, rather than to wither in humiliation and withdrawal. Sturdy, active care and compassion, a mother's contribution to recovery, right hemispheric contributions (Kaplan-Solms & Solms, 2000, p. 198; Schore, 2011) were probably very important in terms of Jill's regaining her capacities and fostering her "stepping right".

PART II

VARIETIES OF COMING ALIVE

Introduction to Part II

In Part II, the focus is more on aspects pertinent to awakenings or processes of coming alive.

Chapter Three suggests that we might be hard-wired by evolution and foetal experience to anticipate a caring environment, as well as other prenatal stirrings, which will shape subsequent experience. The role of implicit (unrecallable) memory in shaping experience is reviewed, as is the role of explicit (conscious) memory with regard to the sense of lived experience.

Chapter Four, as part of the primacy of affect, looks at how much of our reality is really composed of hallucinatory phenomena. It also considers aspects of psychic trauma in terms of affective overwhelm and the crucial role of negation and cortical shaping as part of necessary regulation. The final part of that chapter reconsiders the fundamental nature of hallucinatory experience as a basis of lived experience, but also as primary to identity.

Chapter Five demonstrates how poetry bridges the cognitive and the contemplative, the left- and the right-brain approaches to experience, and strives to illustrate how the metaphoric capacities of the right foster such depth of view.

CHAPTER THREE

Awakenings

*Hard-wiring and preconceptions
as the roots of unconscious fantasy*

R esearch in the past couple of decades is suggesting that the anticipations of a receiving environment and the motivations for relating to that environment are hard-wired at birth. Trevarthen (1996) observes how soon after birth the infant and mother enter into reciprocal gesturing, and, indeed, that the infant reaches toward the mother with the right arm (left hemisphere) and toward himself with the left arm (right hemisphere). He concludes that this is evidence not only of how rich the emotional communication is between mother and neonate from just after birth, but also of significant prenatal organisation. Trevarthen suggests that there is an "Intrinsic Motive Formation (within the limbic system) that emerges in the brain stem at the embryo state before there are any neocortical neurons" (p. 578) and that this formation is guided by the various emotional interchanges which then shape the developing cognitive systems. He suggests that the origins of cortical asymmetry might be due to "the activities of the brain that *precede and anticipate* uptake of information from the environment . . . [such as via] motivation, attention and intention" (p. 571, emphasis added).

Very recent research involving four-dimensional ultrasounds (the added dimension being time) suggests that foetuses can anticipate their own bodily motions, as evidenced by the opening of their mouths to receive their hands at twenty-four weeks of gestation (Ferris, 2015, p. 24). These data suggest that much hard-wiring, or early foetal organisation, anticipates aspects of postnatal development. They echo Bion's conjectures about preconceptions, that is, built in anticipations about unfolding development once the anticipations are met. They also reflect Solms' and Friston's contention that the brain is an intentional, not just a reactive, organ and organiser of experience. It seems that such anticipation, the roots of unconscious fantasy, begins very early in development.

Further observations by Mancia (1981) and Civitarese (2013) about prenatal development emphasise that very early awakenings emerge from the somatic experience of rhythmicity and constancy of the foetal–uterine dyad where all needs are provided and where rhythms of maternal voice and movement and the stirrings from internal organs are part of the milieu. The preferences shown in the neonate for the maternal voice, and, indeed, music heard across the uterine barrier, inform us of the receptivity and registration that is likely to be operating in the later stages of gestation.

In addition, studies (Mancia, 1981, 1989; Schwab et al., 2009) suggest that the foetus, from about seven months of gestation, is engaged mostly in an active REM-type sleep. This underscores Mancia's earlier suggestion that during this type of sleep, beginning in late gestation, there is "a sensory integration tak[ing] place similar to that which occurs in the adult . . . which is the electrophysiological equivalent of the hallucinatory experience of the dream" (Mancia, 1981, pp. 351–352).

He also suggests that this active sleep provides a frame of reference for a primitive nucleus of mental activity, which might foster dream-like activity, that is, REM-type sleep, as well as registering the rhythms and stimuli from the maternal/uterine environment. This nucleus, probably found in the brainstem, matures significantly prior to birth, and might be related to that which Trevarthen refers to as the Intrinsic Motive Formation. These authors might be offering different perspectives about the same thing, although Trevarthen speculates a much earlier state (embryonic) of emergence. Regarding the primitive nucleus of mental activity, Mancia states that its function is to transform the externally derived sensations reaching the foetus during active sleep into "experiences capable of creating internal objects in the form of representations" (1981, p. 353). He suggests that the foetus's intense motor activity, both in waking and sleeping states, could be seen as evacuative of unprocessed sensory–motor elements (Bion's beta elements) (1981, p. 354).

Further, Mancia postulates that the protective functions of the uterine environment, linked with this primary mental nucleus, could comprise a kind of "skin" function which can protect the foetus/baby in its probably violent encounter with the birth process that involves not only the expulsion from the mother's body, but the rapid transformation from a passive intake of oxygen via the placenta to the need for active breathing on the part of the neonate. These beginnings of mental life, as noted by Mancia, then, suggest an outline of somatic experience that gives rise to hallucinatory dream-like phenomena, probably the roots of unconscious fantasy, and the capacity to metabolise sensory into psychic elements (the process Bion terms alpha function).

Mancia's careful considerations about the roots of unconscious fantasy warrant an expansion of contemporary confirmatory views more explicitly discussed in the previous chapter: computational neuroscience (Carhart-Harris & Friston, 2010; Friston, 2010) is suggesting that the brain creates inferences, a concept which goes back to Hermann von Helmholtz, who, in the 1860s, suggested that we have unconscious processes, internally generated from associational learning, to organise and explain our sensory experience. Apparently, Helmholtz was trying to explain why we can get so drawn into a theatre performance, for example, experiencing the gifted young actor as an ancient sage. He postulated that we have unconscious models available which inform our immediate reality (the experience of the performance as the most immediate reality) under the appropriate circumstances. These models act as inferences, ways of organising and explaining the sensory phenomena based on previous experience or expectations. Significantly, these inferences are *internally* generated, and, indeed, in some instances might be innate. Friston's (2010) and Solms' (2013, p. 18) discussions imply that Freud's concepts of unconscious fantasies, as inferences about the world one is experiencing, were probably influenced by Helmholtz's views.

Bion's notions of preconceptions might be heir to this same view. As mentioned previously, the internal inferential models help to structure experience in part by binding free energy. Bion's preconception of the breast, or attentive maternal care, is a good example. Probably a legacy of evolution, it seems that there is an inborn inference that attentive care will be forthcoming. When it is met and confirmed by experience, there is further confirmation about oneself and the world and the inference about good care is strengthened. When the expectation or preconception is *not* met, there might be a jarring dissonance, experienced as deep disappointment in, or perhaps cruelty by, the object. Neurologically, there is a release of destabilising, disturbing free energy. The inference is shaken and recalibrated, and the dissonance might register as psychic trauma. There seems, then, from various perspectives, to be evidence for innate inferences or fantasies that organise experience and intentionalities. Also, when not met and carried forward, these inferences might contribute to disturbances that comprise psychic traumata.

Implicit (unconscious) memory might encode external as well as internal happenings

A subsequent phase in the coming alive of the psyche is that which several authors, including Mancia (2006) and Schore (2011) note as implicit memory. Implicit memory, referred to earlier as registering the earliest non-recallable experiences, is also part of the timeline of emotional and psychic development. In contrast to explicit memory, that which is available to consciousness and has been known about for many years, our understanding of implicit memory has been clarified only more recently.

Implicit memory usually refers to the earlier experiences of life prior to the maturation of the hippocampal structures, which facilitate cortical memory processes, and it is generally believed to be organised by the amygdala. These early experiences date to the last two to three months of foetal life. They are registrations of the prosodic elements, the melodies and rhythms of the mother, her earliest attunements and ministrations. They may be either positive, laying the background of harmony and safety, or they may be negative, registering neglect, trauma, and disharmony. These earliest prelingual experiences are registered in the right hemisphere, where they are likely to remain unavailable for conscious recall. While there are no explicit memories that would support conscious recall available prior to the maturation of the hippocampus at about eighteen months of age, these prosodic elements are carried forward in the individual's voice, bodily expressions, and carriage. The individual's attitude towards, and expectations of, the world may be seen to be written in nearly every gesture in the here and now. When this unremembered, but present-in-the-moment level of experience can be understood and expressed in words and, thus, thought, it can gain the stamp of time and place and, therefore, reside in the past rather than lingeringly haunt the unremembered present of the individual (Schore, 2011). A clinical example might be illustrative.

A while ago, I treated the mother of a baby girl who played incessantly with strings and curtain cords, often wrapping them around her neck. While still a foetus, she was observed via uterine sonogram to be holding the umbilical cord and wrapping it around her neck. This observation, among others, prompted the decision for Caesarean section delivery to avoid the potential hazards of cord strangulation. The baby and subsequent toddler's continued fascination, even seeming obsession, with wrapping the cord around her neck continued until it became disturbing to the mother and became a focus in her therapy. We had realised during her pregnancy that she had intense ambivalence about this baby as a foetus, the pregnancy occurring during a stressful time of her life. But the depth of her negative feelings towards this baby only became more apparent as we thought more about the baby's fascination with strings and cords. As the mother, my patient, became more aware of her hatred of the pregnancy and the baby, more aware of how burdened she felt by her baby amid a precarious marriage, the little girl appeared to play less with the strings and cords. As the mother confronted more openly the difficulties within her marriage and took steps towards the resolution of those tensions, the baby turned away from playing with the cords and took up safer playthings. It is inviting to consider that the baby's playing with the cords echoed her *in utero* playing with the umbilical cord, as responses to some internal signals of distress from the burdened mother. This gesture diminished only when the mother could take more active steps to resolve her tensions, fears, and angers about the marital situation.

This example of gestural transmission across the caesura of birth, but also gesture as an expression of maternal fantasy and emotion conveyed to the foetus, and beyond, might illustrate not only the carrying forward of somatically expressed proto-emotions and fantasies, but the need to appreciate that such gestures, especially regarding hostile, even murderous, fantasies, deserve serious consideration.

In the absence of active recall from the implicit level of experience, it is intriguing to consider that aspects of dreaming, both the unconscious process and the consciously remembered dream, might carry the implicit forward towards explicit recall and understanding.

The work of Mancia (1989) enhances understanding of the organising function of dream-like states in foetal life, and perhaps beyond. From sonographic and neurobiologic studies and measurements of what is considered to be active sleep in the foetus, it seems that, from about six months of gestation, active sleep, akin to REM sleep in the adult, serves an integrative function for sensory input, motor output, and affective (pleasure/pain) learning. Mancia hypothesises that this integration forms a proto-mental nucleus of the self based on bodily experience prior to birth. Such integration serves memory (familiarity with mother's voice and other prosodic elements) and continuity beyond the caesura of birth—all of which enriches the storehouse of experience within implicit memory.

It might not be surprising, then, that remembered dreams can carry forward and represent these implicit memories. Therapists report that dreams can bridge the gap, offering visual and emotional representations of issues that the patient cannot recall, but which "speak" to the heart of early traumatic issues. These dreams probably express aspects of implicit memory and can deeply inform the therapeutic work as well as general efforts involved in growth and development (Andrade, 2007; Joseph, 1992; Mancia, 2006).

A clinical vignette may be helpful.

When I was working with children, I had occasion to hear about their dreams. I have never forgotten that of a sensitive four-year-old boy whom I had the privilege to work with for only a few months, due to his family's changing circumstances. During that time, he made use of play materials, but mostly harnessed his vivid imagination to express and find understanding about his intense feelings about the newly arrived baby sister and his feelings of loss of privilege in the family. On the last day of our work he told me a very moving dream:

He was playing at a sandy beach and had discovered a beautiful blue marble there. But after a very short time he lost the marble in the sand and realised in the dream that he would not be able to find it again until he was sixteen years old.

He seemed to know what the dream meant, and we both seemed moved and sad, which I noted along with the dream's suggestion that the blue marble would be found once again when he was older. That is how the hour and our work ended. I did not hear further how things went for him or his family, but I have frequently thought of our work and especially the richness of that last dream. Admittedly, these are my associations, but my intuition suggested he also had some inkling of the sands of time which would reveal the lost marble, the beautiful marble of the work we had done, but also the marble as the potential for thought and understanding which had not been part of his family pattern. In addition, the dream's message of finding the marble again as an adolescent suggested some forecasting of his wish to find another mind to relate to as we had in our time together, perhaps a wish for that kind of relationship as he moved away from his family into the wider (blue marble) world. Then, and now, I am deeply impressed by the expressive power of this dream, from the imaginative mind of a four-year-old about himself and his future.

Mancia reminds us, further, that the dream provides imagery "able to fill the void of non-representation, representing symbolically experiences that were originally pre-symbolic" (Mancia, 2006, p. 93). In the little boy's dream, there could be several instances of meaningful, even complex, representation: the blue marble of possibly compassionate understanding, briefly found and then lost again until a future date; the need to wait (marble lost in the sands of time) and yet the hope for the future (to be found when he is sixteen years old). These complex representations, of course, might be recognised by the dreamer in an *après coup* form, that is, remembered in a looking back manner, when his symbolising capacities are more mature.

This therapeutic function of the dream is echoed in several authors' observations about the need to access and alter traumatic contents of implicit memory. All emphasise the need to modify the unbound energy and, thus, traumatic affect (Crick & Mitchison, 1983; Freud, 1915e, pp. 190–191, 1920g, p. 19; Hobson, 1994; Winnicott, 1949, pp. 241–247.) The blue marble image might express the beauty and promise of the binding experienced in the brief therapeutic work, as well as the hope for such in the future when the marble can be found again. Andrade (2005) stresses the importance in analysis of the transfer of affect from archaic experiences in implicit memory into the transference experience.

The effect of implicit uncontained affect might include somatic symptoms and fears which appear to have no physical basis in medicine, but which, when sensitively received as communications, might be somatic registrations of gestational trauma and parental inattention. Such implicitly registered traumata might impair explicit encoding and, thus, interfere with the cortical registration that allows a memory to become represented as a thought, and then be put into one's past. When this failure of cortical registration occurs, the trauma remains a potential ever-present torment, such as occurs in post traumatic stress disorders (PTSD).

Andrade (2007) gives a vivid description of a seemingly well-adjusted individual who had a significant history of panic about cardiac collapse, asthma, and other concerns, for which no physical basis could be found. However, when the analyst could shift his attention from interpreting to the well-adjusted demeanour of his patient and instead to give time, space, and attention to these symptoms as communications about something unrecallable, this more open receptivity allowed the gradual revelation of neonatal trauma, which had been poorly understood and addressed. Significant in the successful treatment was the attentiveness of the analyst to these symptoms as communications, which included understanding a dream at the level of the expression of the trauma. Once verbal understanding of the trauma was available, the trauma itself could become part of the patient's past. While not the main focus of Andrade's paper, this sensitive account suggests that when the level of implicit memory can be appreciated as a significant phase of psychic awakening, its contents may become more accessible to the unfolding of lived experience.

Generally, there is a more or less seamless flow between implicit and explicit memory as part of the narrative of one's life. Yet, as Siegel (2012) suggests, unresolved traumatic memories do not become part of the narrative involving the flow of implicit and explicit memory. Instead, they remain like entropic free energy "In an unstable state of potential implicit activations" (p. 79) which might burst upon the ongoing internal experiences of the survivor or his/her interpersonal relationships.

Explicit (conscious) memory registers an experience as lived

In contrast, the products of *explicit*, or conscious, memory become available in the second to third year with hippocampal maturation. The most relevant form of explicit memory for subjective experience is episodic memory (Solms & Turnbull, 2002) or autobiographic memory as stated by Damasio (2010). This form of memory involves the mingling of the two channels of experience noted by Solms. That is, the subjective state from the interior, coupled with the externally sensed events. As Solms and Turnbull state:

> . . . [while] *external events* can be encoded unconsciously . . . (as semantic, perceptual or procedural traces), the episodic *living* of those events apparently cannot. Experiences are not mere traces of past stimuli. Experiences have to be *lived*. It is the *reliving* of an event as an *experience* ("I remember . . .") that necessarily renders it conscious. (p. 161, original emphasis)

Experiences have to be *lived* to become conscious. And the subjective experience of the rememberer, as Solms reminds us, itself initially unconscious, linked with the memory traces of external circumstances, comprises the episodic memory, the lived experience of the ego. The contribution of the interior, subjective state is what brings lived experience to the fore as conscious memory (Solms & Turnbull, 2002, pp. 160–162).

Hans Loewald brings an added perspective: he postulates that in health there is an ongoing dialectic between the products of implicit memory, which he calls primary reality, or primary narcissism, and that of explicit memory, that is, secondary process thought. He suggests that there are two forces in mutual operation: the forces towards unity, merger, and remaining one with the object (i.e., no differentiation) and the second force towards differentiation. These forces are in mutual tension throughout life. For Loewald, the communication with the more highly differentiated mind of the parent aids in the differentiation process, both with the external object or parent and also within the ego and one's own mentation.

Loewald stresses that memory discharged as action rather than represented as thought is coincident with the implicit memory systems, and is the most experience near, while conscious representational (explicit) memory is less so. These two systems are synergistic and co-creating in the to and fro of union and differentiation. All the while, the primary memory requires ongoing contact with parental figures, who help to organise the child's experience toward conscious representation (Singer & Conway, 2011, p. 1191). Where Solms postulates the role of the subjective ("I remember") as vital to conscious memory, Loewald suggests that role comes from parental organisation and is vital to the growth of secondary process (Loewald, 1976, p. 170).

The integrative nature of Loewald's conceptualisations span various theoretical points of view, including drive theory, ego psychology, and object relations:

> [The infant's] relational instinct to be with others and its ego instinct toward differentiation and cognitive complexity work in tandem as the rhythm of its interactions with and withdrawal from objects both propel development of ego differentiation from the object/external world and within the ego/internal world. (Singer & Conway, 2011, p. 1192)

Loewald, similar to Civitarese, describes the harmonious, synergistic interplay of these different elements in growth and development.

But trauma may also be engendered within implicit experience. The range of unconscious processes, which are registered in implicit experiences, allows complex activities to be performed smoothly and efficiently but, because they are automated, that is, out of the range of conscious recall, these unconscious elements are less amenable to change. In terms of their impact on mental functioning, these automated, repetitive patterns often carry intense affect (unbound energy), as exemplified in PTSD reactions. The memory traces of old traumata might then trigger reflexive, undiminished, and, thus, retraumatising responses.

Trauma, which, to a large extent, is registered implicitly, might impair explicit encoding, as well as impede the co-ordination of implicit and explicit memory. The final cortical registration allows a memory to become something in the past. Without this cortical registration, the individual, subject to the implicit experience of trauma, is ever *in* the experience and, thus, not able to *think about* the experience.

Dissociation, which derives from and defends against trauma

may also impair explicit memory for these events in a number of ways by severing the links between memory systems in a way that detaches them from conscious access. The somatic and behavioural aspects etched in implicit memory, however, remain intact. (Pally, 1997, p. 1230)

CHAPTER FOUR

Hallucinatory phenomena

Dreams, preconceptions, projective phenomena, hallucinosis

Hallucinatory phenomena are basic to mental functioning. Bass's notions of the fear of difference (fetishism) and concrete functioning in the face of the narcissistic resistances to difference note their pivotal role. This section will review and expand on some of those understandings. The term hallucination refers to sensory stimuli that arise entirely from internal sources but are generally experienced as coming from the exterior. Solms notes that the precursors of our cognition lie in the affective upwellings triggered by the brainstem, and so all cortical presentations of these manifestations are hallucinatory in origin as they arise from internal sources. For clarity, subsequent cortical *re*-presentations also factor in perceptions from exterior sources, so emerging thoughts as re-presentations might comprise the admixture of hallucinatory (internal) and external perceptual (memory) sources.

Hallucinations seem to provide equilibrating functions in several ways. When the normally active, even noisy-seeming, brain becomes stilled, hallucinations might occur to fill auditory space. Oliver Sacks (2008) cites this and other related phenomena in terms of musical hallucinations filling the void. He notes Hughlings Jackson's observations about release phenomena, that when some higher order (frontal lobe) inhibiting function is impaired, as may occur in stroke or trauma, a lower (temporal or parietal lobe) function, which had been inhibited, is released to function once more. Sacks's examples illustrate the release of musical expressions or talents when the language region has been damaged. This might be a temporary release of the inhibited function, such as in mild resolving stroke, or a more permanent situation of long-lasting impairment (Sacks, 2008, pp. 348–352).

In addition, Friston, Bion, and others suggest that there are implicit inferential models of "how the world is", which shape and give form to perceptions. From Freud onward, important avenues for therapeutic detection of the unrecallable experiences also involve the therapist's resorting to his/her own hallucinatory capacities (Botella, 2014; Civitarese, 2014; Schore, 2011).

Freud's early considerations regarding hallucinations focus on the remembered dream (Freud, 1917d, pp. 232–233). He notes that the remembered dream demonstrates both negative and positive hallucinations. Internally generated visual stimuli (positive hallucinations) are delinked from memory and, thus, from previous experiences and other aspects of external reality. These delinkages, or negative hallucinations, which, in part, protect the sleeper from motoric action, compel the dream to be experienced in terms of intense immediacy, which Freud called perceptual identity (Freud, 1900a, pp. 566–567, 602–603; Bass, 2000, pp. 24–26, 44). That is, "what I see is all that exists and it all exists as 'now'". This understanding also negates any pain or disturbance because, with regard to the mechanisms of the dream, a negative hallucination erases any disturbing internal or external perception. The unconscious registration may persist, but the psyche, perhaps in an effort to reduce free energy, responds as if the perception never occurred. Reality is easily distorted in favour of psychic equilibrium.

Summarising several aspects of his significant work on the negative, André Green (1999) says,

> Hallucination is a representation, essentially unconscious, which is transformed into perception by being transposed outwards . . . It can only be perceived from the outside . . . by passing itself off . . . as a perception, that is, as originating from the outside . . . we are bound to

conclude that wish-fulfillment and primary process tend towards hallucinatory activity . . . (p. 169, reprinted in O'Neil & Akhtar, 2011, p. 86)

Further, Green states that wishful hallucination and perception are so similar that something called "reality-testing" must be postulated to tell them apart. Usually, reality testing holds, but if either the external perception or the internal fantasy is too unbearable, the portion which gives way is perception, and the result is that the negative hallucination prevails (Green, 1999, p. 170; O'Neil & Akhtar, p. 87). He continues,

> Thus negative hallucination is the process by which the ego can break off or interrupt its relations to reality. It can therefore justifiably be considered as the major process which governs relations between reality and the ego . . . (Green, 1999, p. 171; O'Neil & Akhtar, 2011, pp. 87–88)

That thing called "reality testing" appears to be frontal cortex mediation, which aids discernment between hallucination and perception of the external world. Cortical mediation is vital for discerning these various aspects of reality.

There are some interesting correlations between Green's notation and those of Friston about inferences and perception: both acknowledge the hallucinatory underpinnings of perception. If disturbance (free energy) is sufficient, perception is eradicated, giving way to the wish to reduce that disturbance. From his own viewpoint, Green might have been thinking about the same phenomena that Friston describes in his observations about the organism's ongoing efforts to reduce disturbing free energy. What Friston calls inferences, or unconscious fantasies that so shape perception, Green calls wishes that can interrupt the ego's perception of reality.

Students of Bion will recognise Green's formulation of hallucination involving the reversal of the usual mode of perceiving as taking in from external reality. Over his lifetime, Bion (1965) came to view hallucinatory phenomena as a spectrum of projections involving emotions, a position which is similar to that of Solms about affective upwellings entailing specific emotional tones (Panksepp, 2013; Solms, 2013). Following Freud and Klein, Bion felt that the psyche grows through a process of projection and introjection. That is, taking in from the world and projecting outward tensions, but also unmetabolised bits of potential experience to be received and processed by a receptive exterior. Bion also introduced a couple of terms that attempt to describe his complex view of these projective processes: "hallucinosis" is the term he coined for hallucinations in an otherwise intact personality. Hallucinosis might be considered to differ from more elaborated products of the imagination in that, being a hallucination, it is a more sensory-based, reactive response. It is experienced as an unquestioned, concrete given, a kind of "this is how it is, no questions asked", such as occurs in transference phenomena. Thus, hallucinosis lacks the depth of association and potential meaning that products of the imagination generally convey.

The second term, "transformations in hallucinosis", is, according to Paolo Sandler (2015), Bion's attempt to describe a spectrum of responses in the patient when an analyst attempts to bring more psychic truth to bear (p. 1141). The variety of potential responses of the patient comprises the various transformations (changes in form) that he might experience in response to that possibly painful confrontation. For instance, if the patient's response to a revealed pain or truth can be faced, it may stimulate curiosity for further exploration, which would constitute a *transformation of K*, that is, a wish to know more. Another possibility is that the patient may encounter a *transformation of O*, which would manifest as an immersion into an emotional experience, rather than an intellectual insight, following the analyst's interpretative efforts. Other possible transformations along a spectrum of projective transformations involve transference and projective identification. The components of this spectrum of projective transformations are demarcated according to the intensity and violence of the triggered emotion; the more violent the response, the more intense and distorting the projection will be.

Bion also felt that the infant self has innate preconceptions, that is, anticipations ready to be realised in experience. One of the most prominent preconceptions seems to be the anticipation of a caring, metabolising other who will attentively make things better in terms of the baby's projected distress. This function of ordering the world is echoed by Friston's innate inferential models that organise sensory data to give form to our perceptions.

The spectrum of hallucinatory phenomena for Bion, then, involves preconceptions, perhaps having organising functions. When these anticipations of good enough care are met, such as in transformations in K or O, there is a sense of well-being and free energy is minimised. The resulting heightened capacity to bear frustration and delay could lead to space where thinking can develop. However, many times the preconception is not met. This might be due to an unresponsive other mind, or to confrontation with unbearable psychic truth, which feels like an unresponsive, or, indeed, a pain-bringing, other. In either case, the response to pain unsoothed, especially when the expectation has been intense, might be one of profound frustration or disappointment, sufficient, even, to fragment the mind. Such fragmentation might be experienced as one having been abandoned or even betrayed by the object that did not provide what was intensely anticipated.

This intense and destabilising type of projective transformation involves a sudden reversion to concrete experience as a consequence of the collapse of mental space, and the fracturing of one's mental functions.

It might appear to the observer in this situation that the impacted individual has suddenly become concrete and rigid in his thinking and demeanour, while also uncontained, as if lost in space or with thoughts scattered to the wind. But considerations that he has been overwhelmed by intense affective upwellings, as if hit by a tsunami of raw emotion (frustration), are also helpful. Indeed, the patient might seem to spew intense emotion into the mind of the companion or therapist to find a container. The receiver of those spewed emotions might feel that a tsunami has come his way, too. The signature element here is the intensity of the emotion. It is more than the average mind can bear without fracture of some kind. To many, then, this is considered psychotic process, that is, raw, shattering emotion rather than quieter thinking processes. To others (Cimino & Correale, 2005), this range of hallucinatory phenomena, similar to Sandler's view, is considered as a spectrum of violent projective identifications.

Cimino and Correale view the intensity of the onslaught as "unfinished writings" (2005, p. 52) that must be lived before they can be thought about. Once lived, the writings can begin to be finished. Such rescue, in my experience, involves a sensitive mind familiar with this level of emotional intensity that can receive the violently projected shattered bits and aid in completing them as communications. Patience aids recognition of the mental collapse and the preceding rage along with gentle verbalisation of that experience. This reintroduces the anticipated container that then begins to reanimate the debris field, instigating emotional accompaniment and reintroducing mental space for thought. This whole task can be arduous and delicate, requiring the therapist to dip into hallucination as well. Overall, the survival of the mind of the therapist, which includes his ability to stand his ground with regard to his viewpoint, not to just affirm the patient's view, is an important registration for the beleaguered subject.

Less violent forms of projective transformations are those that emanate from a portion of the personality, which again slips into the concrete, perhaps out of terror, guilt, or rage around a circumscribed situation. These situations do not fracture the entire mental apparatus, but do cause distortion within a sector of it. Again, the aspect of the mind focused on the problem succumbs to the intensity of the pain-bringing emotions and allows that intensity to define reality. To the subject, then, this concrete reality feels absolute and his projections might feel like "intensely conveying my clear view", but to the receiver the intensity and concreteness of those projections might feel like penetrating missiles in a takeover bid for one's mind.

An example, similar to my previously cited vignette (see Chapter One, pp. 19–20), would be when outrage arising within a narcissisti-cally vulnerable state of mind insists upon precise affirmation, and experiences any non-affirmation to be a sudden loss of the affirming object. This jarring loss is felt as "being mean" or "causing me pain". Critical here, again, is the sturdiness of the receiving mind, that is, its being able to receive the shards and temporarily experience their violence. Striving to find the potential messages that triggered the outrage begins to restore the object felt to be lost and, thus, also begins the task of reconstructing mental space and thought.

Another example of this less violent hallucinatory situation, which can still captivate a certain sector of the mind is the mental state often termed a conviction. Here, the individual feels certain that he/she has unique access to the "truth" about a situation and also looks down contemptuously upon all others, as if no one else has a clue as to the reality that the conviction conveys. While this stance is again fuelled by intense, concrete certainties or saturated preconceptions amid an otherwise intact personality, it can still hold the rest of the personality in thrall.

A clinical example: a patient with a somewhat obsessive disposi-tion, fearing his wishful fantasies about embezzling funds from his workplace, became increasingly convinced that his fantasies had become reality and, thus, would be noticed by the auditors at his firm. These fantasies became more and more fixed, despite repeated discreet discussions with the auditors, who felt certain that nothing amiss had occurred in the firm's finances. My patient developed the conviction that his view was correct and that the auditors and senior management were wrong. Only he knew the dreaded "truth".

Of course, he also became contemptuous of me, his long-time analyst, as I tried gently to explore the nature of this entrapping conviction. Only when I could allow myself to feel into the guilt and terror that had become his reality, as well as his dread about his fantasy becoming the unassailable "truth" about himself as an embezzler, could I begin to speak to the grip of the conviction. When I could slowly and carefully offer comments such as "how terrified and guilty he felt . . . feeling certain that he deeply deserved to be found out and prosecuted for his intense fantasies . . . and certain no one else could understand that gripping dread and the depth of his guilt . . ." could he feel some welcome relief and release from the conviction. I believe my being able personally to appreciate and then speak to the depth of the terror and dread was important in reaching him and helping to bind that terror into thought. The imagery came to mind of him becoming frozen by the terror into concretely experiencing the intense emotions as unassailable "truths". These images arose from my reading Bion's notations (1957, 1967) as a compass, which aided my search for this man so encased within in this dread-filled conviction.

Of course, my patient's conviction was also fuelled by his feeling of internal fraudulence or embezzlement, that is, the draining of his internal resources and offering lies in the place of painful truths. I found in the clinical work that the conviction about the external embezzlement precluded his being able to think with me about the internal situation. It was not until we could address his terror of being found out in the external world that we could then address the ongoing internal disturbance. It felt that he needed to experience my capacity to become an emotional ally rather than a judging auditor before he could do so as well. In Cimino and Correale's view, my patient might have needed my "finishing the writing" regarding the viewing of terror and dread from an empathic rather than a persecuting stance before he could emerge from the conviction sufficiently so that we could then proceed to the next level of mutual understanding.

The least violent of the projective transformations are those seen in transference manifestations: we expect in the future what we have experienced in the past. These expectations shape current perceptions and lived experience. These projections mostly involve the reality of the projecting subject, his/her sense that the transference is reality, although those upon whom the transference is being projected might sense something a bit askew from the distorted emotional responses embedded in the transference.

Interestingly, the intensities which lead to the collapse of mental space and the accompanying reversion to the concrete provide a clinical picture similar to that which Solms describes, especially in patients with lesions to the right associational cortex. These lesions interfere with healthy functioning that fosters visio–spatial cognition. That is, the subject's orientation to external physical space and to internal mental space as well. (Kaplan-Solms & Solms, 2000; Solms &Turnbull, 2002). So, it might be that the explosion and collapse of mental space caused by intolerance of frustration or intense, concrete emotion correlates with structural switching off of this level of cortical processing. The violent shards might be the now unmediated affective upwellings, experienced as missiles to the previously cognitively organised mind. The flattened concrete debris field might be the inner experience when mental space is collapsed or absent. The potential for metaphoric transformation, such as my patient's rescue from the conviction, is only available when mental space and understanding are restored. My patient seemed able to regain that space by internalising that understanding. Unfortunately, for patients with right associational cortical lesions, according to Kaplan-Solms and Solms, such understanding and insight might last only for the duration of the therapist's physical presence.

Civitarese (2015) describes how the analyst's attempt to rescue the patient gripped by hallucinosis requires the analyst's loosening his or her ties to external reality. Following Bion's advice, the analyst deliberately attempts to divest himself of the products of memory and desire, that is, contact with the cortical cognitive functions. This step facilitates regression to the level of his encumbered patient and perhaps, via mirror neuronal functioning, to resonate with that unverbalisable pain. This function, as described by both Bion and Civitarese, is not a violent act, as described with one who succumbs to frustration intolerance. It is an action that is more measured, suggesting that cortical mediation is not entirely switched off. But this level of hallucinosis is of value only when the analyst can subsequently "wake up" and re-engage his dreaming, symbolising self to be able to think about the just experienced pain.

This use of hallucinosis, as cited in the vignette about conviction, operates as a rescue mission, dipping into the well of the inexpressible but then reconnecting with potential thought. This description of hallucinosis might be thought of as cleaving the union of the input from the external world with its links to the past (memory) and the future (desire) in order to venture via resonance and mirroring towards the wordless, affective upwellings with their intrinsic emotions. Solms' notation that these interior upwellings must be linked with cognition for recognition and representation would be what the waking up, as described by Civitarese (2015), would accomplish.

It is interesting to consider that Bion's dreaming and the transformation of the concrete involves the right hemispheric contributions of imagery and mental space along with the verbal symbolic functions of the left associational cortex, all sent forward to the prefrontal cortex, which reconnects these aspects with the affective upwellings to reconsolidate the core sense of a conscious self. Solms and Turnbull (2002) note that the function of the prefrontal cortex is a close correlate of the functions of maternal reverie, that needed object, which can apparently cause such frustration. Transformations in hallucinosis may, then, be thought of as both the violent destroyer of the link with the needed object as well as offering the initial steps towards rescue of the mind, which needs reunification with that object.

The deepest anxieties might be hallucinatory eruptions

Solms emphasises that we have a narrow tolerance for disturbances to our inner sense of well-being. When those narrow limits are exceeded, our affective responses might lead to an eruption of varying intensity, including the terrifying *tsunami* of undifferentiated affect that Bion termed "nameless dread" and Matte-Blanco (1988) referred to as the "sweep of symmetry". The terror here comes from the "namelessness" that occurs as the inner self is swamped by some archaic, anonymous, eruptive force. Solms clarified that these internal arousals need to be registered and represented by cortical work to become detectible to our conscious selves. He succinctly states this is what has to occur in order to quell the terror or dread. For the rescuing mind to function, these disturbing arousals must be received, registered, and represented as images and words. That is, the waves of terrifying affect need to be made into "mental solids" (Solms, 2013, p. 12). This is done by the cortical processes, which are the inscriptions of that experience, the "waves into objects" that cortical, environmental containment provides.

Do the basic anxieties of the fear of death that Freud and Klein postulated derive from experience that leaves the individual feeling an anxiety that is far more intense than signal anxiety? An anxiety that is a "helpless[ness] in the face of overwhelming stimulus" (Freud) or with a "disintegrated mind" (Klein)? Although Freud and Klein each seem to view this primary anxiety slightly differently, as Blass (2014) suggests:

> both find the source of primary anxiety in a state of disintegration and loss of a potential for psychic response. For Freud, this takes the form of being helplessly stimulated in the face of loss; for Klein it is the disintegration of the mind. (p. 624)

In a careful examination of Freud's and Klein's views of the fear of death, Blass states that for Freud this fear is of the

> state of being overwhelmed by stimulation without there being present any coherent sense of self that could do something with this stimulation . . . [while] Klein's fear of death rests . . . on a range of experiences associated *with the death of the mind, which emerge, when in phantasy, the self is destroyed.* (p. 623, original emphasis)

As both of these states may be the result of a *tsunami* of untransformed affect, it might be unifying to consider that such is one, if not the major, cause of the fear of death, the terror of annihilation, the dread of the dissolution of one's capacity to think. In addition, if unmediated affect is the primary internal source of annihilation, the death instinct could be envisioned along a spectrum from biological surrender, or passively giving up the fight, to the ego's actively throwing itself into the de-differentiating maelstrom.

A sense of self, of subjectivity, then, is based on hallucinatory experience, that is, sensory experiences arising from internal sources.

Affects, which are ever-present, provide the background template for the subjective self, even being the page upon which experience is inscribed (Solms, 2013, p. 7). As well, these upwellings pose a potential psychic trauma, which can be dealt with by binding the energy in words and thoughts. There are other means of handling these energies as well.

Varieties of response to traumatic affect: dissociation, disavowal, projective identification

Disavowal in which opposing attitudes are kept separate, but accessible via shifting identifications, has been discussed at length in our consideration of fetishism (Bass, 2000) and will not be repeated here.

Dissociation may be defined in a number of ways: many psychoanalysts compare and contrast dissociation and projective identification as two manifestations of the splitting processes. Dissociation is cleavage, considered less violent in nature and remaining primarily within the individual, with the self losing touch with its own agency. Projective identification is often described as the more violent cleavage of unwanted aspects of the self, which are then projected into external objects, both for riddance, but also in order to control the target of those projections. Dissociation is also described as an attempt to contort the self in order to be acceptable to, or identify with, usually parental objects. The irony is that the attempt to maintain union or harmony always leads, as does projective identification, to impoverishment of the now fractured self. Once the mind has been split, there is almost always a reversion to concrete states of mind, due at least in part to the collapse of mental space and the attendant cleavage of the capacities for symbolic thought. With every regression or reversion, destabilising free energy is liberated.

While all engage in dissociation, such as becoming lost amid fantasies or entertainments, more persistent dissociation might occur when the personality has been exposed to trauma or severe developmental strain. Dissociation may derive from the parasympathetic system's inhibiting capacities that operate in dialectic opposition to the sympathetic arousal mechanisms (Schore, 2002, p. 451). In these instances, the generally integrated emotional and cognitive patterns that comprise lived experience are disrupted, and one loses one's sense of agency: that is, "who I am". Dissociation has been described as a form of splitting in which reality imposes a split of the ego (Blass, 2015, p. 125).

Neuroscientist Heather Berlin (2011) writes that dissociation can be defined as "a disruption in the usually integrated functions of consciousness, memory, identity or perceptions . . ." (p. 16).

When dissociation more completely defines the personality it may be considered as depersonalisation disorder (DPD), which Berlin describes as

> a dissociative disorder characterized by a persistent or recurrent feeling of being detached from one's mental processes or body, accompanied by a sense of unfamiliarity/unreality and hypo-emotionality, but with intact reality testing. (Berlin, 2011, pp. 16–17)

She offers a detailed description of the neural underpinnings of dissociation, which include several mechanisms, such as the cortico–limbic disconnection hypothesis. This suggests that diversion of attention, a frontal lobe function, can deactivate or numb the sense of a coherent "who I am", that is, of the subjective self.

She also presents findings (2011, pp. 17–19) that suggest at least two distinctly different subjective states of "who I am" can be registered simultaneously. Dissociated identity disorder (DID), the most complex form of dissociation, usually triggered by childhood trauma, may include significantly different identity states with distinct neurological and other physical registrations for each state.

> Physiologic differences across identity states in DID also include differences in dominant handedness (which may indicate opposing hemispheric control of different identity states), response to the same medication, allergic sensitivities, endocrine function, and optical variables such as variability in visual acuity, refraction, oculomotor status, visual field, color vision, corneal curvature, pupil size, and intraocular pressure in the various DID identity states, compared to healthy controls . . ..

She describes a patient with DID who, after years of psychotherapy, had some resolution of cortical blindness. One startling aspect observed in this patient was that

... visual evoked potentials were absent in the blind personality states, but normal and stable in the sighted ones. .... This case shows that, in response to personality changes, *the brain has the ability to prevent early visual processing and consequently obstruct conscious visual processing at the cortical level.* (Berlin, 2011, p. 17, my emphasis, added to highlight how the body can be impacted by, and respond to, traumatic experience)

These data suggest that the mechanisms that impose a split on the ego (Blass, 2015, p. 125) might create significantly different physiological responses in the different identity states within the same individual. As well, the case of the cortical blindness which seemed to resolve somewhat with therapy might illustrate the ego's attempt to fend off, to become blind to, the various penetrating traumata, and only be able to resolve the blindness when the deeper trauma were tended to therapeutically: that is, to be seen by a receptive mind.

Berlin mentions that the diagnostic categories of psychiatric dissociation and neurological disconnection syndromes appear very similar. Following her significant review of the literature on neurological investigations of dissociative disorders, her summary thoughts include the following:

What appears to be altered in both neurological disconnection syndromes and dissociative disorders is not so much the degree of *activity* of a brain area or psychic function, but the degree of *interactivity* between such areas or functions. Integration of various cortical and subcortical areas appears to be necessary for cohesive conscious experience. (2011, pp. 18–19, original emphasis)

Here is further evidence of the vital function of the cortical interactivity and its function in the binding of free (traumatising) energy. Apparent as well is the potential consequence, that is, dissociation, when such integrative binding is not in place.

Several authors have written about the analyst's well-intentioned efforts being traumatic, even violent, to a patient. Herbert Rosenfeld (1987) sensitively considers how the analyst may become traumatised by the patient's volatility, or snagged by countertransference issues. Without sufficient self-analysis, the therapist might then reactively retraumatise the patient, creating a potential impasse in the therapeutic work. Rosenfeld's work alerted a generation of therapists and analysts to the need for sensitivity and tact in interpretative work with vulnerable individuals.

Michael Diamond (in press) reminds us that a secondary dissociation may come into play when the dissociated individual enters a therapeutic situation. The original fracturing trauma that impaired the neural mechanisms of the coherent self can be compounded by insufficient understanding of the dissociative dynamics, which will inevitably occur in the therapeutic situation. He suggests that an initial task of the therapist is to validate the emotional trauma of the patient in terms of introducing the function of a validating mind. Then, it is necessary to anticipate the patient's both reliving in the transference the original trauma, as well as re-enacting with the therapist the would-be protective dissociative manoeuvres. Diamond suggests that recovery from dissociation inevitably involves the repetition of the trauma in the process of its transformation into understanding. As in hallucination or violent projective identification, this calls for the therapist to be able to bear the slings and arrows of the trauma as the traumatised individual does to the therapist what was done to him/her. Once again, the survival of the therapist's sturdy mind, so vital for transformation of the trauma into understanding, means that the therapist must survive, and both verbally and empathically express what the patient experienced and is now enacting transferentially. At the same time, the therapist must maintain his/her separate viewpoint. Empathically verbal representation in an atmosphere of sturdiness and respect offers repair to the injured associational cortices. The patient needs distance from the traumatising experience to begin to think about, rather than be trapped by, emotions, and defined by the trauma itself.

This aspect of repair, noted by nearly all authors cited regarding the treatment of psychic trauma, might also address what Ferenczi has noted in the trauma of absence. That is, parental neglect, for whatever reason, is felt by the nascent self to be abandonment, leading to the self-definition of "only worthy of being abandoned or attacked". Ferenczi's "absence within an absence" suggests strongly the anticipation of care and protection gone awry. When the anticipation of care is not met, the self feels defined by the abject sense of abandonment (Gurevich, 2008).

These ongoing references to the rescuing mind, and the seeking of such even amid the ravages of considerable psychic trauma, echo

Bion's preconception of in-born searching for the receptive mind. In cases of dissociation, it is possible that what goes awry is this innate expectation not being fulfilled.

Clinically, then, the deeply dissociated individual, such as in dissociative identity disorder (DID), might present with very provocative, seductive, or aggressive behaviour, often defensive, but still catching the therapist off guard. While the external view might appear as if the individual is fully aware of his/her provocative behaviour, from an internal view, that is, in terms of the inscriptions on implicit memory and, thus, automatic behaviour, the provocation could indeed reveal the degree of traumatic experience the deeply dissociated individual might have been exposed to. Solms (2013) and Friston (2010) might suggest that, in these circumstances, the traumatic unmediated affect (free energy) fails to be securely bound and, thus, secure the child's early experience. In Bion's terms, the preconception for care has been negatively realised. The carers have traumatised rather than comforted their child. Parenting figures who lie, distort, or blame the child for being traumatised have set the scene for provocative behaviour to be repeated with the therapist. The seductive, deceptive, contemptuous-seeming dissociated individual might have been caught up in an automatic repetition of the deeply wounding, frightening, overwhelming unbound affect he/she has had to bear. His/her own shattered inner world, where excitement, seduction, and contempt replicate the trauma experienced, also attempt to defend against the abject humiliation experienced by the traumatised person.

Due to the intensity of the presenting behaviour in the consulting room, these scarred people can be experienced as intentionally contemptuous and seductive. Their sense of agency having been obstructed, they are automatically repeating the trauma and belittlement they themselves felt when unprotected and exploited.

The dissociative experience might, then, be considered the best the patient could do in managing the betrayals and affective assaults of a traumatising environment. The various bits and pieces of the self harbour various aspects of unbearable affect, including the initial abusing contempt toward the would-be rescuing therapist. The whole mind of the therapist is needed to bear the fear, excitement, and panic which had so traumatised the patient as a child and to validate and re-authorise the patient's sense of self and agency.

Projective identification, already discussed in terms of hallucinatory phenomena and unbearable narcissistic distress, is understood from a variety of perspectives. For London Kleinians, "there is a tacit assumption that 'projection' and 'projective identification' mean the same thing, and that 'projective identification' is an enrichment or extension of Freud's concept of 'projection" (Spillius et al., 2011, p. 126).

Additionally, ". . . the distinction is based on retaining 'contact' (with the contents projected) in the case of projective identification and losing it in projection" (Spillius et al., 2011, p. 142).

Cimino and Correale (2005) suggest that the intense form of projective identification has a violent intrusive impact on the receiving mind. It can feel like a bolt from the blue which overwhelms his/her separately thinking mind, and

> hark(ens) back to traumatic contents of experience coming from . . . (implicit) non-declarative memory (p. 55) . . . They [the violent affects received] are made of inert fragments of psychic material, [debris from the violence of the trauma], that are felt rather than thought (p. 51) . . . [and thus are best considered] not as unconscious contents to be revealed, but rather as writing to be completed [by a receptive mind] (p. 55)

Cimino and Correale cite the automaticity of such penetrating projective identifications as one of the hallmarks of both the power and the unconscious nature of these emanations from the projector. Very probably, the power of the projection mirrors the power of the originally experienced trauma or accrued traumata registered in implicit memory and projected into the here and now as a transference manifestation. They cite the importance of the "writing to be completed", but also what a strain this is on the receiving mind.

While not addressing the violence and trauma but, rather, the wider phenomena of projective identification, Pally (2010), citing shared emotional circuitry and mirror neurons, offers the view that projective identification may be considered as the relationship to mirror neuron functioning. The analyst can automatically resonate with the patient's emotional state, even the disowned affect from the patient. In addition, Schore (2011) refers to projective identification as involving the right-to-right brain communication, which bypasses conscious mediation to bring penetrating emotion into play as an influence, if not a weapon.

Referring back to Green's mention that perception gives way when mental processes are under too much strain,

> . . . the portion which gives way is perception, and the result is that the negative hallucination prevails . . . Thus negative hallucination is the process by which the ego can break off or interrupt its relations to reality. It can therefore justifiably be considered as the major process which governs relations between reality and the ego . . . (Green, 1999, pp. 170–171; O'Neil & Akhtar, 2011, pp. 87–88)

At face value, this statement suggests that negative hallucination, the erasure of the products of perception, governs reality for the ego. Bion, whose work was deeply admired by Green (1992), would probably offer a slight amendment, suggesting that the degree to which the preconception of good enough care is realised governs the ego's relationship to reality. Both of these positions echo human and, perhaps, mammalian experience. Among mammals, there might be evolutionary preconceptions or anticipations for maternal care to help one make sense of the chaotic-seeming internal and external world. Also, if there is substantial neglect, overwhelming stress or trauma, there might be complete reversion to survival, rather than to care. Both pathways may be inscribed in evolutionary legacy.

Under duress, such as when our ancestors were being chased by the lion or when modern selves are pursued by internal fears, neural responses will bypass the deliberate thinking processes provided by cortical input and (re)turn instead to the more archaic, rapid, reactive responses of subcortical circuits. The amygdala and hypothalamus circuitry triggered by fear or unmodulated affect kick in here. This reversion to more primary modes of defence is in complete affirmation of Hughlings Jackson's contention that "dissolution of higher order (neural) centres would encourage the re-emergence of lower level functions" (Feinberg, 2010, p. 149). While life saving for our ancestral selves, the consequence of this reversion to subcortical circuits is that it closes down the option for the more evolutionarily recent experience of time and space for thought and transformation of that affect. Instead, we are cast (back) into the frenzied, pressured mental world of concrete functioning, good, perhaps, for staying on the run from the lion, but less adaptive for managing our inner uprisings.

The potential of our pre-thinking evolutionary past, in terms of innate expectations that alter aspects of current reality, can be further observed in Bass's (2000) notations about fetishism and his explorations of the dread of difference and differentiation in concrete states of mind. When the need to erase the awareness of differentiation, with its ambiguities, goes beyond what is bearable, the individual reverts to the hallucinatory state of the dream mechanisms. Perceptual identity and temporal immediacy create a state of mind which embraces firmly bounded opposing fantasies of "all good" and "all bad", and rigidly held "certainties" of "friend" and "foe" as all of reality. The self locked in this position could form a hard shell of certainty or conviction to ward off the painful vulnerability. A group, a belief, or a tribe may be adhered to for security, not daring to be open to uncertainty and change.

It is noteworthy that these defences of negation, and the previous considerations of various splitting mechanisms, involve reversion to the concrete: that is, the turning away from cortical input that would maintain the link with complex reality, including dreads about difference and uncertainty. These defensive regressions to more primitive functioning utilise massive denial of the aspects of reality that the psyche cannot bear to deal with by reverting to the subcortical route of the ancients.

While these states might feel like clinical pathology, it is important to realise these hallucinatory aspects are employed in daily life. Firm edges or boundaries that are basically hallucinatory are taken on to secure one's sense of identity, one's tribe, values, or ideals. The degree of rigidity needed to hold on to these everyday hallucinatory creations probably relies on one's relative comfort with hovering doubt: the more doubt about one's identity, values, or even mortality, while still maintaining one's capacities for reflective thought, the less rigidity one would require. The less doubt that can be borne, the more rigid, even to the point of conviction, one miught have to become. Doubt as an agent of de-animation, in terms of triggering entropic free energy, might be a useful metaphor.

The pressures toward de-animation bring the edges of disappointment, disillusionment, and despair into view regularly, owing to the incursions of doubt and uncertainty. Whenever one, as analyst, feels fatigued, distracted, or otherwise out of touch with a patient or one's therapeutic self, a measure of de-animation (entropy) sets in. At the best of times, the self-assurance about firm boundaries, self-knowledge, and sturdy working capacities are hallucinatory phenomena, which stem from an internal sense of well-being (Solms, 2013) and psychic integration. As important as these hallucinatory self-assurances are regarding establishing inner space and linking with reflective capacities, being hallucinatory in origin, they are subject to erosion whenever one's inner sense of well-being is altered.

For example, with sufficient doubt, due to my own distraction, fatigue, or a penetrating accusation from my despairing patient, my sense of live-minded, reflective thought can be significantly eroded, perhaps even to the point of collapsing into a sense of hopelessness or paralysis. The rescue from this deadened state requires the re-animation of my self-reflective capacity so that I may observe my situation as one of temporary erosion rather then just being swept away into the conviction of paralysed helplessness. The revitalisation of self-reflection reinstates my appreciation of the limits of my humanity and, indeed, the capacity to contemplate my disappointment or despair as states of mind rather than as catastrophes. However, when the forces of entropic de-animation take hold, that self-reflective function and its rescuing capacity are lost, and the spectre of becoming entangled in a perpetual helpless collapse reasserts itself.

To live is to appreciate the need to strive and to differentiate so that we can observe and evolve in our thoughts and creativity. Yet, to live is also to recognise that our sense of who we are and how well we are functioning is an ever-present hallucination, which leaves us continually vulnerable to the sweep toward de-differentiation.

*   *   *

While it is challenging to consider that we live largely amid our hallucinations, it might make it easier to understand the madness of human violence. The splitting which creates the hallucinatory work of "who I am and what I know" can also become polarised into good and bad, my tribe and the other/enemy. These strongly held polarised positions, cleaved by the violence of the splitting mechanisms, become the only realities available to the mind steeped in this black-and-white world. Operating, then, on the level of the jungle mentality, there is no reflective thought at all available to this state of mind; all is action, impulse, doing what one is told. The atrocities of the twentieth century (and, of course, other centuries as well) might be more explicable when viewed from this awareness of the hallucinatory world. Conviction, but also the tyrannical hold of the power-based left-brain function as parts of this reality, might also aid in explaining the intransigence of this state of mind to rational thought. While not uncontroversial, Milgram's experiments on obedience to authority (Milgram, 1974), and Zimbardo's Stanford Prison experiment (Zimbardo, 2007), demonstrate how readily one's own authority and sense of self may be surrendered amid external coercion, or the illusion of power as an authority, offering illustration of our vulnerability to this jungle mentality and to these aspects of tyranny.

* * *

A personal dream specimen illustrating the more benign spectrum of hallucinatory functioning concludes this chapter.

As I was thrashing about with the writing of this chapter on hallucinations, focusing intently, trying to synchronise one author's thoughts about the dream with those of another, I felt at times a kind of futility, as if I had been too closely focused on dream mechanisms and so had lost the wider view of the forest, as it were, my left cerebral hemisphere functions eclipsing those of my right.

That evening I had a dream.

> I was to introduce a presenter at a seminar, someone who was a colleague of mine, and I had been worried about divulging that detail in the introduction, although it was fine with the presenter, who had given me a short introductory text. Waiting for the seminar to begin, I realised I was in a dark, empty room at the appointed time, so I walked out to look for the seminar leader and presenter and entered a well-lit room, replete with food and drink and full of lively people. That room had a graciously curved bar in front of the food, in some contrast to the rectangular, beige, empty-seeming room I had been waiting in previously.

I awoke, feeling a bit drab and restless until I let the associations of my struggle with detail from the day before associate with the drab, dark, empty room of the dream. Immediately, I felt energised to think about the dream as a communication rather than a condemnation, that it could be understood as referring to the state of mind in which I had felt entrapped in the dream, rather than a definition of who I was as a drab, colourless person in reality.

A few things came to mind:

- that the image in the dream as a hallucination was "what I see is all there is", that is, that I was drab and lifeless, but when I could let memory link up to the image, I could see more deeply; I could shift from being defined as drab to viewing the dream and feeling it as symbolic of my previous day's struggle. This seemed like a good illustration of what occurs when memory and thought can be linked with the dream image: it gains dimension, and becomes a representation of an experience rather than a total judgemental definition. I could now view below the surface, beyond the drab, empty room to see the representation of an experience I had had. Here, then, the hallucinatory "truth" transformed into a meaningful symbol about an emotional experience was something I could then think more fully about as more associations came into view.

- I could also see the presence of condensation, splitting, and idealisation in the dream: my disappointment in my previous day's writing efforts, not up to the standard I had hoped, had been condensed in the dream to a beige, empty room. In addition, splitting had created an idealised situation in the dream where all the light and life was outside of the room, while I was in the dark. That darkness had initially defined my mood upon waking—my feeling drab. But as I could ponder the dream, seeing through the surface into the depths, and perhaps allowing some of the fruits of my previous day's writing struggle to come to mind, I could view the dream as illustrating the very things I had been trying to write about. That is, the hallucinatory phenomena of upwellings of slight disturbance (the disturbingly beige and empty room), the reversion to splitting into images of dark and light, and the need for the seeing through the surface to the depths for the real insight. Once I could see these elements, I felt the hallucinatory experience had been transformed into meaningful information and I was grateful for the light and enrichment of the dream.

Perhaps as a companion piece, but also to offer contrast, here is an example of what I would call bedtime hallucinosis: when, for bedtime reading, I look at the current *Science* or *Scientific American* magazines, trying to decipher the latest micro-biological or cosmic discoveries, reaching far beyond what I can really grasp at this hour of the night, let alone this time of my life, I am indulging in the hallucinosis that I can really embrace and understand these far-reaching insights. I strain to learn but, in fact, probably in this over-reach, I fatigue my much smaller sphere of reasonable grasp, whether that is, perhaps, the scope of this book or my recent thoughts about certain patient dilemmas. This hallucinosis (noted by Bion and others as a hallucination in an otherwise intact personality) has to do with the recognition of the reasonable boundaries of my mental, perhaps emotional, reach, *vs.* the reach of my fantasy of boundless capacity.

The rescue from this hallucinatory state would be the more modest honesty about my reality, which would involve my ceasing to grasp for those "insights" that will always lie beyond my reasonable reach. I may choose to remain in awe about the boundlessness of the cosmos, but it is best that I stay content with my capacities, humble in my endeavours and, thus, be able to feel nourished by my own experience. And to realise that the dazzle of the inaccessible "insight" is actually a veiled attempt to avoid the reality of my human limits and limitations.

The neural underpinnings of my hallucinosis (Bion's term for a hallucination in an otherwise intact personality) may be complex, but we might be able to view the disconnection from the mutual influence of right and left hemispheric functions. Most basic might be the spatial dimension of the right associational cortex, which, when disrupted, leads to either the collapse of space and subsequent narcissistic entrapment (Solms' description of the right hemispheric syndrome) or the sense of getting lost in space. Without reliable inner space and a sense of personal boundaries to house self-reflective thought, I am subject to the confabulations spun by my untethered left hemisphere in its musings about my boundless capacity. My realistic looking at myself, seeing through the hallucinosis to the more modest reality, is the co-ordinated view of right and left, as when necessary bounded space is available to allow the fruits of self-reflection.

CHAPTER FIVE

Hovering at the interface between mental worlds

M ost of our waking life is spent in the world of the explicit: language based, detail orientated, ruled by the everyday schedule of the waking world, where we are involved with things to do and places to go. This world of appearance, analysis, and achievement is vital to our identity and relatedness in the external world. It is also, more or less, how our western achievement-orientated culture works, at least on the surface, where our consciously perceived and functional efforts measure who we are and how we are in the world and within our communities. This way of perceiving, functioning, and grasping reality is that registered and propagated primarily by the left cerebral hemispheric functions, which deal with language, differentiation, and detail.

Musings upon awakening at dawn

If we look a little deeper, we might glimpse another mode of perception and engagement, that relevant to the less conscious right hemispheric functions. On occasion, just as we are awakening from sleep, we have access to the unconscious world we are emerging from with its evanescent imagery, its shadows, its potential new thoughts which feel soft, but possibly far reaching, while we are also becoming increasingly aware of the awakening world bathed in brighter light, tending toward sharp edges and crisp, word-based language. Verbal language and daytime thought cannot capture the imagistic, non-linear "logic" of the dream, or the essence of the kaleidoscopic, fathomless region of this enfolded mental and emotional realm. This is where poetry helps out, because this world of the dream and the shadow needs symbols and language to make it recallable and thinkable to us for registration in memory and for our conscious analysis. The experience of hovering at the interface between the implicit and explicit worlds might be like watching the level where water and oil meet. Often, our experiences just upon awakening allow us to see both sides of the divide, and perhaps, thereby, to have more access to the implicit than during the bright light of daily activity. Residing at this interface, we may gently glimpse, and, likewise, gently struggle, to find a symbol or a word to capture the sense as contrasted to the full clarity of our experience. An example of such an experience is trying quietly, upon awakening, to remember a fading dream. Poetry often comes to our aid in this endeavour. Hovering at the interface, it offers a view of the interpenetration of these two ways of being.

The explicit "light of day", then, labels "who I am" by way of my actions and productions in the external, consciously perceived world, while the implicit enfolds the many flickering possibilities that comprise a network of hidden memories and registrations, which remain unconscious most of the time. These implicit elements might, however, come forward quietly, as does the remembered dream or the created poem, or they might come piercingly into awareness, as do transferences and other hallucinatory phenomena from amid the multi-faceted strands of unconsciously represented and unrepresented states of mind.

Poetic considerations in the opening up and the closing down of the mind and the heart

This musing at dawn illustrates the interface between the implicit and the explicit aspects of experience, a stance that characterises much of poetry.

Several aspects of poetry addressed by McGilchrist (2009) may be seen in this just-stated reverie:

> We need to see *through* the eye, through the image, past the surface: there is a fatal tendency for the eye to replace the depth of reality . . . with a planar re-presentation, that is, a picture. In doing so, the sublime becomes merely picturesque. (p. 373, original emphasis)

Looking "through the eye . . . past the surface" exemplifies that position of awakening at the interface, where we may quietly try to capture the fading dream.

McGilchrist suggests that the poetic position, similar to Virgil's presence for the Pilgrim in Dante's *Inferno* (Hollander & Hollander, 2000), offers guidance towards self-discovery via the ever-deepening circles of experience. This seeing past the surface refreshes the flattened experience, which often accompanies the bright light of everyday language and assumption.

Scheler suggests that the enigmatic dream world, with its emerging forms, also expands, as does poetry, our capacities for experience and self-awareness (McGilchrist, pp. 341–342).

Also, being at the interface might also illustrate Wordsworth's perceptions that "We *half* create and *half* perceive the world we inhabit" (McGilchrist, p. 369, original emphasis). Wordsworth reminds us, as does Winnicott (1960), but also Friston and Solms, that from this position reality is both created and perceived as a reciprocal process between perception and expectation, between what senses declare and what our minds create from memory and from inevitable hallucinatory dreams and fantasies.

Lingering at the interface, seeing both sides of the divide also suggests not foreclosing with a too rapid rush towards meaning, as this closes down the evolutions of experience in the moment. Staying open to perceive the fading dream might invite open-ended associations, while trying to rush to capture the "meaning" of the dream as part of the busyness of the day, would shut down space for further emergences.

Goethe's view of the deeper perception of reality revealing it as an ever-evolving process, echoes Loewald, Bass, and Hegel's perspectives: "The phenomenon [reality] must never be thought of as finished or complete . . . but rather as evolving, growing and in many ways as something yet to be determined" (McGilchrist, 2009, p. 360; also p. 507, fn 44).

Witnessing the complexity of the unconscious realms, birthplace of our dreams and our dreads, brings us face to face with a realm that is so much more encompassing than our conscious selves can fathom. In this way, we may experience awe and the sublime. Compelling natural surroundings, whether external or internal, can invite one to step aside from the personal pressures and breathe in the slower pace of the wider reality. That is, to find unity with something greater than oneself. In so doing, one might then feel more open to a poetic stance, a relaxed, non-judgemental curiosity. Such an atmosphere then allows one to be receptive to, rather than judging of, others' viewpoints, and to trust in the emerging dialogue, not as absolute truths, but as the emerging associations that can offer creative new ideas. This kind of encounter fosters respectful sharing among all ages and levels of experience. It may soften inner dialogue, the tendency to be harsh or critical towards emerging processes. Heidegger's philosophical considerations of being-in-the-world as fundamentally linked to wide-ranging care (1996, pp. 53, 54) echoes this realisation.

McGilchrist also cites a riveting example of what a poet can instigate in terms of the shift in cultural values, in this instance from the values of the Enlightenment, which included order, stasis, and rationality, paired with the minimisation of ambiguity and metaphor, towards those values of Romanticism representing the ongoing depth of human experience. He says

> ... the post-Enlightenment world was reinvigorated ... by its recursion to the Renaissance, particularly by the rediscovery of Shakespeare, a vital element in the evolution of Romanticism ... It yielded evidence of something so powerful that it simply swept away Enlightenment principles before it, as inauthentic [and] untenable in the face of experience. It was not just his grandeur, his unpredictability, and his faithfulness to nature that commended him. In Shakespeare, tragedy is no longer the result of a fatal flaw or error: time and again it lies in a clash between two ways of being in the world or looking at the world, neither of which has to be mistaken. In Shakespeare tragedy is in fact the result of the coming together of opposites. (McGilchrist, p. 355)

This passage describes how bringing opposites together in an artful way adds power and depth to experience, rendering the intellectual values of the Enlightenment as less authentic, less true to lived experience. This engagement of opposite trends, with its resulting turbulence, might lead to internal evolutions:

> In tragedy, we see for the first time in the history of the West the power of empathy, as we watch not just the painful moulding of the will, and of the soul, of men and women (the constant theme of tragedy is *hubris*), but the gods themselves in evolution, moving from their instincts for vengeance and retributory justice towards compassion and reconciliation. (McGilchrist, 2009, p. 272)

McGilchrist, in this latter extract, poetically addresses the pain, which attends the shift from vengeance towards compassion, and from retribution towards reconciliation—the basic shift from left-brain to right-brain values.

He suggests that reality has a depth and nuance that our everyday eyes and minds can miss when attuned to immediate action and to what is encountered on the surface. Living amid a busy, demanding world pressures one to act quickly with apparent clarity and certainty. Bass's reference to a "defensive counter-surface" is an example of both the "surface" and the "certainty". We develop carapaces, which aim to reduce our anxiety about uncertainty. As we cling to these shields, these hallucinated "certainties", we avoid the sublime aspect and the terrors of the depths.

Put slightly differently, in his notations about the poets and the evolution of ways of being, McGilchrist captures the essence of one struggle faced by all. Being drawn to the familiar offers comfort and apparent clarity, but also avoids the pain of uncertainty and complexity. Remaining open to depth and to the sublime requires an active effort to not form a protective carapace, or a defensive counter-surface comprising an unquestioned certainty or truth. Remaining open invites doubt and uncertainty, both of which can feel erosive (Bass, 2000). This might bring us closer to the heart of "becoming": remaining open to learn and to grow, while also protecting and closing oneself as needed for digestion, continuity, and identity. Can poetry illuminate other aspects of experience?

In a recent book, *The God of the Left Hemisphere* (Tweedy, 2012), Roderick Tweedy brings to attention some interesting considerations about the left hemisphere's qualities of disengagement from emotion and its pressing its agenda towards power and control. He finds substantial verification of these qualities in the poetry of William Blake. As a Romantic poet and artist, Blake (1757–1827) wrote in the period following the Enlightenment, whose values of unimpeachable reason were being countered with the return to the lessons from emotion and the body. In several long poetic works, Blake portrayed "Urizen" ("your reason"), which we would think of as left hemispheric function, to gain God-like status *in its own eyes*, purely by its capacities of division, abstraction and categorisation.

One of Tweedy's main emphases is similar to Bolte Taylor's view that "the emergence of left-brain dominance was the emergence of a *personality*" (Tweedy, 2012, p. 39, original emphasis). And significantly, this reason-based personality is more interested in ruling than in care and concern. It can be viewed as tyrannical or demonic, easily leaving its host to suffer all manner of pain and delusion rather than to admit its way of viewing the world is other than the best show in town.

Tweedy reminds us that it is the very capacities of the left hemisphere that contribute to this demonic power: ". . . the capacity to abstract one thing from another, to compare and contrast, define and describe . . . to separate and delineate night from day, light from dark . . ." (2012, p. 15) can seem to the emerging mind to be dictating to the cosmos.

He suggests that the left hemisphere, in viewing itself as a Creator, Urizen, considers that "before" its emergence and domination, "existence was, or appeared to be, Chaotic" (2012, p. 34). What hubris, we may say, that the left hemisphere might declare itself God. But Tweedy's discussion offers compelling thought about this possibility. In addition, he suggests that the story-telling qualities of the left-brain are the spin doctors of creation myths. Quoting Plato:

> God therefore, wishing that all things should be good, and so far as possible nothing be imperfect, and finding the visible universe in a state not of rest but of inharmonious and disorderly motion, reduced it to order from disorder, as he judged that order was in every way better. (Plato, 1965, p. 42)

Here, "disorder" would be a right hemisphere view while the God (left hemisphere) declares its products, that is, "order", as much preferred.

From a neuroscience perspective, the omnipotent–omniscient God of Reason can be seen to have evolved from the omnipotent sweep of uncontained affective upwelling, its terrifying sweep (entropic free energy) triggering the defensive development of a rigid, inhibiting counterforce. The usually balanced right- and left-brain send their products forward for the fontal lobes to re-present and to sequence for thought-based reflection. However, this powerful frontal lobe function might become hijacked out of terror of that potential upwelling, and, thus, suspicious of all affect. In this situation, the intellectual left-brain becomes a self-described omnipotent Emissary (McGilchrist's book title is *The Master and his Emissary*) and convinces itself that it has subjugated the original Master, even labelling that primal energy as the chaos, which has to be ordered.

Interestingly, then, the myth of creation may be read as derision for the right hemisphere as being the "chaos and formless infinite" from which order is extracted and, thus, goodness is imposed. Tweedy further cites Blake's references to Urizen's psychopathic tendency towards cruelty, brutishness, and, again, self-elevation when it is split off from, perhaps even contemptuous of, psychic pain and human emotion:

> Thou knowest that the Spectre is in Every Man insane brutish
> Deformd that I am thus a revening devouring lust continually
> Craving & devouring
> > (Blake, "The Four Zoas",
> > vii: 36–38, in Erdman,1988, p. 360)

Recalling the character of Richard III in Shakespeare's play, Blake specifically draws attention to the divided nature of what he calls Rationality, the separation from emotion and empathy that compels one towards control and domination and points out that this division needs to be confronted and recognised before any meaningful reintegration can occur.

> The Spectre is the Reasoning Power in Man . . .
> An Abstract objecting power, that Negatives every thing
> This the Spectre of Man, the Holy Reasoning Power
> And in its Holiness is closed the Abomination of Desolation.
> > (Blake, "Jerusalem", 10:13–16,
> > in Erdman, 1988, p. 15)

Captured in a few lines (Jerusalem 10:13–16) is the negating, the objecting to everything which typifies the doubt-ridden, close-minded state of negation, but also the arrogance ("Holiness") of those who hold themselves superior to others' views. This aspect of a divided mind is caught up with power and possession. Dissociated as it is from the living, breathing aspect of being alive, it turns toward domination and possession of things but, always feeling unsatisfied in its alienation, it may, thus, become inflamed by greed, envy, and material acquisition.

Tweedy describes the reversion to concreteness (falling from Paradise) and the self-damnation or imprisonment of the mind that occurs when greed and envy are uncontained. I have chosen to quote this portion of Tweedy's book because we will revisit the fall, as depicted in Milton's *Paradise Lost*, from another view in Chapter Six.

> The "hardening" process or "damnation" as Milton calls it—is the central psychological process of [his monumental poem] *Paradise Lost*. Satan's trajectory of "falling" . . . is in part a counterpoint to the loss of paradise itself. And as Satan falls [his view becomes "hardened" or concrete, and literal] . . . *Paradise Lost* thereby depicts the gradual process of self-damnation in Milton's most memorable and dramatic character, the state that Blake also refers to as "Satan". (Tweedy, 2012, p. 241)

Tweedy shows us that Blake wisely demarcates individuals from states of mind in his consideration of Satan. He suggests the satanic state of mind (that motivated by greed and envy) is one that can be fallen into, but also emerged from. Satan, Adam, Eve, and other biblical characters can be imagined as literal persons rather than as states of mind. Envisioning them as states of mind offers more hope, more of a sense of movement through difficulties, rather than of being caught forever. Re-envisioning the processive view, as seen in most of the authors reviewed, provides the more integrated human view of reality.

To recall, from a different source, with the power of this division of minds, how persuasive the left brain can be, here is a quote from Jill Bolte Taylor, whose unique experience of observing and recovering from a left-hemispheric stroke provides vivid evidence of the power of the left-hemispheric functions:

> when I experienced the haemorrhage and lost my left hemisphere language centre cells that defined my *self*, those cells could no longer

inhibit the cells of my right mind. As a result, I have gained a clear delineation of the two very distinct characters cohabiting my cranium. (Bolte Taylor, 2008a, p. 133, original emphasis)

Bolte Taylor could witness the distinctive characters, the different qualities of mind, and could give witness to the dominating power of language. This is in alignment with Solms, who describes the powerful role of words, which transform waves of affect into mental solids that can be thought about. But thoughts can become truths rather then remain mediated waves of affect; this is understandable, for we are thinking creatures, *Homo Sapiens*, "wise, rational man", who pride ourselves on being able to dominate our environment and to conquer the unknown via thought. Such pride, however, can make us lose touch with how distorting this capacity for thought can be when it alienates us from the more sensuously based, right-brained self.

Significantly, Solms (2013) and other neuroscientists cite the inhibiting function of the left hemisphere, suggesting that the whole of the cortex inhibits and modulates the affective upwellings. McGilchrist (2009) also mentions that, in isolation, the left hemisphere confabulates. It makes up stories to explain what it does not know: "my brother's arm", the left brain rapidly mentions. The patient with a right-hemisphere stroke (and, thus, now mainly functioning with an isolated left hemisphere) is confronted with the paralysed arm that it wishes to dismiss or to disavow.[7] The left brain names, but it cannot see below the surface of the current circumstance to assess context, which might include significant loss. Left-hemispheric functions appear to block out suffering by disavowal and confabulation. This is a picture also seen when right cortical damage erases the sense of bounded space. Only when there is integration with right-hemispheric functions can the left hemisphere then (re)gain contact not only with context, but with emotion, so that it may express and experience care and pain about losing a part of oneself to stroke or injury.

The complex issues involved are glimpsed when the dominating tendency of language, thought, and belief are allowed to overshadow the quieter, but more intuitive, wisdom of the embedded, integrated self. Integration seems to involve awareness of this wider, complex situation, which requires a "casting off" of the mantle of left-hemispheric domination.

Blake contends:

Each Man is in his Spectre's power
Untill the arrival of that hour
When his Humanity awake
And cast his Spectre into the Lake
(Blake, "Jerusalem", 41, in Erdman, 1988)

Tweedy notes about these lines,

Blake writes this enigmatic and powerful quatrain in reverse hand-
writing ... Perhaps this suggests that man is not ready to read this
writing, or that in order to read it one must look at things in a slightly
different way, as it were, back to front. One must "awake": from the
state of what is normally called "consciousness", but which is also a
profound state of unconsciousness, of sleep-walking ... McGilchrist
also characterizes the rational, "conscious" left hemisphere as an
insouciant sleepwalker, walking towards the abyss. Only ... by
becoming *aware* of these false and destructive drives ... can the individual truly awake. (Tweedy, 2012, pp. 265–266, original emphasis)

I offer this long extract from Tweedy's book because the theme of
"sleepwalking" and being warned to "wake up" are also mentioned
by Solms (2013, p. 14). The cortical functions that approximate Freud's
ego aim at automaticity. That is, to make conscious attention to various functions unnecessary because those functions, as they become
familiar, can be carried out by subcortical and, thus, unconscious
mechanisms (2013, p. 14). Solms, thus, suggests that the aim of the ego
is towards sleepwalking or towards becoming a zombie. In other
words, towards making consciousness *un*necessary. This idea, as
noted in a first reading of Solms' "The conscious id" (2013), felt stunning to consider there. Yet, encountering it again after reading Tweedy
and Blake, one can see that the depiction of domination by a ruthless
Urizen is a kind of sleepwalking state in terms of the turning away
from the pains, sufferings, and joys of lived experience.

Returning to Blake's poetic resolution, that is, the confrontation
with Urizen and reintegration of it with right-hemispheric qualities,
Tweedy notes,

But perhaps Blake's greatest achievement in presenting this process of
awakening and confronting the [left-dominated] Selfhood, is his poem
Milton, which re-enacts this moment of confrontation between the

poetic principle, or "human Imagination" [here, "Milton"] and the inurements and enticements of the Selfhood ["Satan"] . . .

In Blake's poem the figure "Milton" comes to . . . [the] realisation that it is *his own mind that has set up the potency of "Satan"* . . . what has to be cast out, therefore is not "Satan" but one's [obstructive] Self . . . [via] Self realisation. (Tweedy, pp. 268–269, my emphasis)

The casting out means recognition of that which allows disengagement from the god-like enthralment, as defined by the satanic constraints and certainties. Psychoanalytically, we understand this disengagement to involve emotional insight and emergence from the frozen constraints of the narcissistic point of view. That is, being able to see what felt like the absolute, frozen, unchanging reality as one of several possible states. From an external view, this realisation appears smooth and easily accomplished, as does the transition from bud to flower to fruit. The process appears seamless, even elegant. However, the *internal* recognition that precedes the disengagement witnesses turbulence in this process and, thus, the need for sturdiness to discern the frozen constraints as products of brutal division, rather than as unassailable "truths". To have these aspects seen, for the divided self, feels like brutal scrutiny. Blake, in this passage, intimates as much with terms such as "annihilation" and "smite" suggesting violence, indeed destruction.

Taking half a step back, the origin of this frozen inhumanity, this disengaged world, which Blake captures so poetically, can be viewed from Hegel's position as initially the externalisation of disturbance in order to get to know it. This externalisation impels the self to view that disturbance from a position of the examining eye, perceiving and insisting that such disturbance is "outside" the self. Reintegration involves the repatriation of that disturbance as part of self. This process means realising that not only the obstructing disturbances, but also the divisive forces that aim to disown the disturbances, are not external. Such recognition, indeed, annihilates the myth of being the power at the centre of the world, and re-establishes the more humble processive to and fro involved in learning. In lived experience, this clear view and dismantling of omnipotence is not a gentle process. It is one that involves bearing pain and tension as one softens the hardened carapace, risking feeling humiliated, as one owns the disavowed elements, before feeling the relief of reunion.

In the lived moment, that pain and tension involve the risk of embracing need, which has been felt as weakness, trust taking the place of cynicism, attentive care seen as other than manipulation or domination. As mentioned, this reunification process might involve a jarring and then disarming shift from power to the wider awareness of vulnerability and need, as humiliation trends toward humility. McGilchrist might say that the left-hemispheric values yield to those of the right, but the subsequent inflow of softening gratitude and insight, which accompanies a reunification of the fractured self, is often interrupted by sudden reversions to the old polarised positions. This phenomenon, known to clinicians as a negative therapeutic reaction (NTR) (Anzieu, 1986; Olinick, 1970), is a testament to the resistance to change and the power of the familiar. The resistances to change can seemingly erase the hard-won integrative efforts in a few moments. To the externally observing clinician, it can be a breathtaking experience to witness the instantaneous erasure of the emotional integration, insight, and mutuality which accompany integrative work. But such erasure makes more sense as we recall that integration, as in all living processes, means "swimming up-stream" against the ever-present entropic pressures which would otherwise sweep one towards de-differentiation and decay. To the patient who experiences the NTR, it is as if the previous integrative work never occurred. There seems to be the possibility, possibly via a negative hallucination, of a total annihilation of recently gained emotional insight and memory. Change, then, in terms of emotional integration and insight, often requires repeated consolidating experience, while also appreciating the ever-hovering allure and occasional return to past polarised and entrenched states of mind.

The results of this reintegrative effort are poetically conveyed by Tweedy as he describes Blake's vision of this reunited psychic world:

> ... Urizenic rationality, instead of controlling, dictating to and "using" imagination, now becomes imagination's vizier and protector. It is imagination that now wields the enormous and enormously beautiful function of science. Once man uses reason, rather than Reason using man, the reintegration of the hemispheres is realised. (Tweedy, 2012, p. 290)

To annihilate oneself for others' good, then, involves the surrender of the products of dominating thought to the intuitive processes of the embodied self. This rather monumental task for the power-based self requires trust and faith, a paradigm shift, which we shall address further in the Chapter Six.

Music as an integrating language of the body

Another form of the poetic in terms of its depth and reach into our emotional experience is music. While not a specific focus in this book, it certainly deserves attention in terms of its capacity to have an impact on lived experience. Being so linked with the body and its rhythms, music speaks the language of the body, potentially rich with emotion, even into the unrememberable past, as it may trigger the primordial rhythms and other soothings first experienced *in utero*. Also, because of its bodily connection, the types of memories and sensibilities linked with music might outlast other types of memory, which are more language based (Sacks, 2008, p. 380).

McGilchrist notes the importance of music and its ancient origins and he observes that lesion studies underscore the intimate link of music with primarily right-hemispheric functions. Left temporal lesions, which reduce one's capacity for language, might not involve one's musical appreciation and abilities at all. Such lesions in the right hemisphere obliterate those musical capacities nearly entirely (Sacks, 2008, pp. 74–75).

As well, there have been many reports of autistic and other individuals who might have difficulty with spoken language and emotional engagement to become much more expressive when encouraged to sing their communications (Sacks, 2008, p. 234, fn). Once again, the capacities to reach beyond the immediate, into the spaces afforded by poetry and music, aid the blocked and the fearful aspects of our experience.

A deeply psychotic patient of mine found that when she was especially tormented by traumatic memories and (now internalised) voices, various styles of music could help to calm these anguishes. Part of our work involved thoughtful consideration of her associations to these various soothing musical forms and artists, each of which was linked with deep emotional expression and, thus, a quieting containment. Her link with music was a significant aspect of our therapeutic work.

PART III
BECOMING AND BEING

Introduction to Part III

This concluding Part reviews other aspects of lived experience, including the courage to face the turbulence of our authentic emotions, our "being conscious" rather than holding to the shield of "thinking we are conscious" (Solms, 2013).

CHAPTER SIX

Becoming: the continuing process of coming alive

We half observe and half create the world

The wisdom of lived experience gathers strands from various sources—neuroscience, philosophy, psychoanalysis, history, literature—each enriching our understanding about what transforms the inanimate into the animate, what occurs in awakenings, in coming alive.

Neuroscience emphasises how primary affect is for all of neural functioning, but also how vital is its mediation by cortical processes in order to enable consciousness of those affects and their intensities and valences. These cortical processes, noted as the left-brain functions of cognition, include language, detail, and, indeed, the internal divisions, which give rise to a sense of a separate self. However, the products of language and thought, so prominent in everyday lives, can coerce one into believing that thought-based products, rather than affect, are the most trustworthy portals into reality, growth, and transformation.

Memory is prominent in shaping perception, as stated by Solms and Turnbull (2002):

We all automatically reconstruct the reality we perceive from models we have stored in our memories . . . We adults *project* our expectations

... onto the world all the time, and in this way we largely construct rather than perceive ... the world around us. ... (Solms & Turnbull, 2002, p. 155, original emphasis)

An elegant and humorous example of our seeing only what we expect to see is ensconced in the now famous video of the person in the gorilla suit walking across the basketball court, and being unseen by the about half of the observers tasked with tracking ball-handling details (Simon & Chabris, 1999). In an updated version (theinvisible-gorilla.com, 2010), for those familiar with the gorilla's appearance, the change of colour of the background and a player leaving the scene during the video offer renewed reminders that we only see what we anticipate.

Dialectics is key to a processive approach to reality.

The dialectical process, which Hegel and others suggest, lies at the base of all of physical biology and psychic growth (Mills, 1996, 2000, 2002; Ogden, 1992a,b, 2002). This process transcends personal boundaries, and, as individuals, we surrender entirely to the process, as do the cells involved in the transformation of the bud to the flower to the fruit. In the interweaving of thoughts, the giving and receiving, a "shared operation of which neither of us is the creator" is formed (Merleau-Ponty, 1945, p. 354). This surrendering process dissolves personal boundaries if narcissistic tendencies do not obstruct the to and fro. Personally held perspectives fade from view as deeper common ground becomes revealed. The emergence of significant creativity amid a non-authoritarian atmosphere, attested to in Chapter Seven, might be an example of this deeper common ground. Several authors consider that an emerging discussion from such common ground is what arises in true dialogue (Giegerich et al., 2005, p. 5; Ogden, 1994, p. 1; Reis, 1999).

The poetic state of mind sees beyond the surface towards the depth, unless the eye becomes fastened to the surface, or to the glitter of excitement, flattening the potential depth and emergent meaning into a concrete representation. McGilchrist offers glimpses of poetic insights, which enlarge everyday views so as to "extend the scope of our possible self-awareness" (McGilchrist, 2009, p. 342).

Blake's depiction of Urizen ("your reason") is seen as the closing down of the mind, in its efforts toward domination and power. Milton's *Paradise Lost* sees the same process of closure in Satan's fall, as a consequence of his rebellion against a God he refused to worship. As Tweedy mentions,

> The "hardening" process or "damnation" as Milton calls it—is the central psychological process of *Paradise Lost*. . . . As Satan falls and hardens, so Eden is viewed as further and further away . . . *Paradise Lost* thereby depicts the gradual process of self-damnation in Milton's most memorable and dramatic character, the state that Blake also refers to as "Satan". (Tweedy, 2012, p. 241)

The fall, then, away from Paradise, might be seen as the sweep back into concretisation. That is, the hardening into the absolute which once again imprisons, sheering off realisations of choice, and space for reflective thought and the recognition of goodness.

But the fall might also be seen as the departure from the god of the absolute, daring to become the modern man who questions, rebels, and discovers his own individuality. While *Paradise Lost* has often been seen from the perspective which values the adherence to the perfection of the Garden of Eden, it may also be read from the view of the explorer who dares to leave this paradise. As Chuster (2014) suggests, the medieval Christian world seems to have depicted eating the apple of knowledge as the sin of hubris. That is, going against the dictates of the absolute god, daring to explore and to think on one's own as worthy of expulsion from Paradise, and, indeed, subject to the Inquisition, which declares independent thought as heresy. From the modern secular perspective, being seduced by the snake to eat of the fruits of knowledge would be seen as the first explorations into separation, following one's curiosity, the first "no" to the perceived external authority. The snake as insinuation, calling one to go against the rules of the Garden, is interesting and deserves more thought.

In either case, there is a fall from "grace", that is, a being cast away from the comforting certainty into uncertainty, where dread and doubt prevail. The medieval world, from a Christian view, was one of certainties, whether of heaven, hell, or purgatory. The modern secular world is more one of uncertainty, as man contemplates infinities, whether of the external cosmos, or the internal unconscious world. Uncertainty is inevitably accompanied by doubt and its darker companion, dread, both of which are part of the experience of modern man, who might then quest, even nostalgically, after the fantasied, dread-free certainties of the unquestioned Garden.

As moderns, we are invited into another kind of grace, that of dialogue with its offerings of receptivity, learning, and change. However, our narcissistic proclivities still hold us back, declaring the value of certainties as to who we are, what we believe, and the importance of our firmly held identities which must not be disturbed.

Through the lens of the medieval view, eating from the tree of knowledge is the betrayal of unquestioning obedience, which includes the suppression of curiosity. Through the lens of modern man, the fall may be viewed as the consequence of daring to step away from the unquestionable known, in exercising one's curiosity and taking responsibility for one's actions and choices. Growth of the mind is possible here, but not without the dreads of isolation and vulnerability. Such a fall could then be seen as daring to emerge from the encapsulation of narcissism and its pure, eternal, paradisiacal surround into the unknowable universe with all its doubts and dreads. Such a step is transformative for the growing self (Chuster, 2014, pp. 178–180).

This metaphor of the fall from Paradise is actually useful when trying to think about the turbulence experienced in most emotional explorations. A musing of my own might serve to illustrate this.

When I am passionately investigating a topic, hoping for understanding, being unsure where the search will lead, I will be likely, time and again, to ask "Is this the way?" And each search, while falling short of the goal, might offer some illumination or an additional direction to explore. To make use of these new possibilities, I must manage the hovering doubt that accompanies such explorations. This means maintaining inner access to the awareness that such doubt is a manageable worry, rather than evidence of a catastrophic error or hellish condemnation (the fall from Paradise) for having questioned the certainty of the known. If I can maintain this inner barricade against the erosive effects of doubt and uncertainty, I might appreciate the cumulative fruits of these searches, which include a growing appreciation of the unfolding complexity triggered by my quest.

A reminder, once again, that, at our edges of knowing, the ever-present allure of concretisation hovers. It seems that we trend towards the concrete in much of our thinking, especially when we may be even slightly overreaching the limits of our grasp of a subject. This can be exemplified in the statement by a notable physicist, regarding an idea that becomes distorted and misused due to its being concretised into an object (Dyson, 2015):

... Erwin Schrodinger invented wave functions as a way to describe the behaviour of atoms and other small objects. According to the rules of quantum mechanics, the motions of objects are unpredictable. The wave function tells us only the probabilities of the possible motions. When an object is observed, the observer sees where it is and the uncertainty of the motion disappears. Knowledge removes uncertainty. There is no mystery here.

Unfortunately, people writing about quantum mechanics often use the phrase "collapse of the wave function" to describe what happens when an object is observed. This phrase gives a misleading idea that the wave function itself is a physical object. A physical object can collapse when it bumps into an obstacle. But a wave function cannot be a physical object. A wave function is a description of a probability, and a probability is a statement of ignorance. Ignorance is not a physical object, and neither is a wave function. When new knowledge displaces ignorance, the wave function does not collapse; it merely becomes irrelevant. (p. 73)

This statement might illustrate a couple of significant issues: first, a state of mind which has sufficient grasp of the subject (a noted physicist viewing wave functions as probabilities illustrating ignorance) to resist concretising the idea of a wave function into an object, while also clarifying how concretisation can distort: "ignorance is not a physical object, and neither is a wave function ... when new knowledge displaces ignorance the wave function does not collapse; it ... becomes irrelevant". In addition, this statement illustrates how our usually visual efforts to create metaphors (probabilities as waves) might easily lead to a concrete image (the wave collapsing into a single point), which we then believe. Dyson, I think, beautifully illustrates, here, how our ignorance can lead us towards clinging to our images as concrete, solid things to hold on to and believe. Another example of the products of thought distorting in a manner that makes us feel that "what we see" (the image of a wave and a pinpoint) is all of reality.

In psychoanalysis, as well, we tend to concretise clinical data into scenarios or narratives and then to believe these constructions. It is difficult not to, because it is hard to listen with evenly hovering attention as Freud advised (Freud, 1912e) to allow the references to underlying issues cohere for a moment and then de-cohere again. Having faith that there will be creative cycles of coherence and de-coherence in the emergence of unconscious processes is a strain when we are faced with uncertainty and the wish to find clarity for our patients and for ourselves.

From impatience amid doubt to patience amid awe (Bion's Transformations in K and O)

Thus, when I can be genuinely open to the confusions and distractions that inevitably accompany these explorations, I might allow myself to feel, but not be overwhelmed by, the attendant doubts (not collapsing from the fall from certainty). I am then taking the necessary steps towards the sculpting of new internal space—space that reveals the complexities not only of the uncertain external reality, which remains hidden from superficial views, but also complexities about the internal realities honed by my efforts. My initial zeal and impatience in the face of doubt and uncertainty, with proper attention and careful mediation, will be very likely to give way to a patience and humility born of suffering and endurance of the encountered tensions and frustrations. These experiences might yield the greatest fruits of the whole endeavour, for patience and humility, amid faith in the value of the overall project, sculpt an inner space that fosters quiet reflection amid awe—not another paradise or return to the all-providing womb, but a contemplative space which fosters the ongoing emergence of unfolding depth and richness. This opening of the mind via the *expansion of inner space* can then be viewed as the path towards the deeper reaches of reality.

The trajectory of Bion's contributions to thinking and becoming illustrate this sojourn. Students of Bion (Civitarese, 2013, 2015; Ogden, 2004; Sandler, 2005; Vermote, 2011) identify an "early Bion" and a "late Bion" that demarcate different emphases in his explorations towards psychic truth. "Early Bion" refers to his focus on the transformation of sensory experience into meaning and thought via a function well illustrated by the sensitive mother receiving the sensory disturbances that her infant cannot bear to feel. The baby's cries or discharges of these unbearable tensions are taken in by the mother, who tries to get to know them so as to make them bearable and even meaningful to her infant. This process of getting to know, described by Bion as K (for Knowledge), involves the mother's rhythmic, attuned, intuitive responses, which bring her baby in touch with the vitalising aspects of those discharged tensions. Alpha function, then, which is Bion's term for this reverie process, might involve the sculpting, shielding transformations towards being vitalised rather than being overwhelmed by the undifferentiated aspects of reality, which might confront and confound the fragile psyche. It may be parallel to Hegel's externalisation of disturbance for examination prior to reintrojection as a bearable part of self. A significant difference, however, would be that the emotional experience offered by the maternal reception—a sense of being cared for—might have become installed in evolution as a prenatal anticipation that, when met, gives rise to the sense of being recognised and affirmed, another aspect of coming alive. Such an evolutionary anticipation, noted as a preconception by Bion, is one element, which, when realised via experience, gives rise to satisfaction, affirmation, and growth. Trevarthen's Intrinsic Motive Formation (1996) and Mancia's considerations on prenatal development (1981), and the emphasis on the inference as vital for internal harmony and growth (Friston, 2010), align with this view.

Alpha function, then, is at the heart of the process Bion describes as container–contained. This process embraces both the receiving function of the reverie (the container) and the at times overwhelming tensions or affects derived from lived experience (the contained). It involves both conscious and unconscious processing and remains one of dialectical tension, container and contained being mutually dependent upon one another.

Coming alive to our lived experience, in Bion's thinking, requires such a mutually dependent process. This way of working, transforming sensory experience into thought via reverie, occupied several years of his working life and is referred to as Early Bion by his students.

However, in his later work, he began to feel that language, the usual vehicle of thought, might obstruct the emergence of soft-edged intuitions and dream-like images and experiences. He was, in these later years, interested in the interface where the undifferentiated (termed "O" by Bion) takes on finite and, thus, representable form, "at the interface" between the world of the dream and that of the bright light of day, where right-hemispheric functions yield to left-brain representations, that is, at the point where thoughts emerge.[8] Vermote (2011) suggests that in looking toward the undifferentiated emerging into thinkable form (a transformation of O to K, in Bion's terms) one would perceive the emergence of something new, which differs from "early Bion's" concern about the processing and thinking about existing emotional experience (Vermote, 2011, p. 1091). This earlier transformation of sensory elements into images and then thoughts required tolerating frustration until a cohering image adequately represents the previously dispersed elements. Late Bion requires a background of patience and trust that "entails (the attitude) of waiting and tolerating doubt and mystery until something finite emerges from infinity" (Vermote, 2011, p. 1092). Trust and faith are necessary states of mind in these "late Bion" formulations.

A vignette from my own clinical experience might illustrate some of these issues. A while ago, I seemed to be in the midst of musings that would spontaneously occur during or just after rather intense emotional experiences, as if to give form to those experiences so that I might further think about or understand them. One such musing from the consultation room follows.

> The startle of recognition that the "problem" at hand for my patient at this moment is a person I suddenly realise is someone I know rather well but in an entirely different context. My first impulse is to defend this other person, who seems to be such a target of rancour. But this descent into what would become mutual harangue would close me off to a deeper understanding of my patient. So, I actively seek the wider perspective of listening to my patient's here and now concerns, wherein the "problem" might be a realistic concern for my patient, while also becoming both a screen for his/her projections, and one of several possible views of a complex situation.

> In trying to attain this wider view, a feeling and then an image seem to come to my rescue. In the midst of my patient's intense complaints and aware of my different relationship to the person who is currently felt to be such a problem, a feeling arises of being amid differing realities, discrete but connected in some deep way. And then comes an aerial image of several local islands and their surrounding, connecting sea. The image is calming because it seems to offer a sturdy representation of the discrepant views about the "problem" as different aspects of the same reality. The tension of different realities is resolved when I can apprehend the image of different aspects (islands) of the same reality. It seems that the capacity for varying imagery and distance in terms of the mind's eye is key to being able to navigate these shifting views of reality with a reasonable, compassionate compass.

Associations to this musing: this visual image and the spontaneous widening of the field served to absorb my feeling of startle and the intensity of "complaint" about the "problem at hand" for my patient of the moment. In a way, the visual was both a container and contained in Bion's sense. The image of an aerial view of separate islands connected by a surrounding sea represented the distinctly different realities I was experiencing, while also offering the context of the deeper connection (the surrounding sea). My experience was that this imagery allowed both the intensity of my patient's complaint and of my startled, potentially defensive, emotion to be contained by offering the context of multiple simultaneous realities or emotions (several islands). And it felt as if the gently emerging nature of this image fostered this containment. Indeed, I live and work near a marine environment (Puget Sound, where there are many islands), an environment which could give form to the emergence. This perspective suggests a "transformation in K", in Bion's terms, the cohering of various alpha elements or dream thoughts into a pattern, offering space and potentially meaningful thought.

But this vignette might also be considered a "transformation of O to K". The undifferentiated realm of the immediacy of my patient's intense complaint and my startled defensive impulse gives way to the emerging imagery and subsequent thought. This might exemplify the "point where the undifferentiated gets a finite form, a point in infinity where he/she could see the thoughts as they emerge" (Vermote, 2011, p. 1115). Also, it could be considered as an example of what Bion termed the "language of achievement" (Sandler, 2005, pp. 391–397): a finite representation with roots in the infinite or undifferentiated realm (Vermote, 2011, p. 1114), a clear image that has mediated the intense (infinite) "certainties" of the complaint (and my impulse towards a defensive response). The representation (the image) itself seems to have brought added dimension to my experience and perception of the situation of my patient, but it also fostered my appreciation of the wider situation, which is not constrained by my patient's intensities. I believe that the potentially frozen, fixedly certain complaint, which had gripped my patient (and me for a moment in my defensiveness), was dissolved for me by the image. Or, from a slightly different angle, the imagery, in allowing a way forward so that I could view my patient's intensities as one of several realities, offered the mental and emotional space needed for my transformation and growth.

This example might demonstrate how impatience amid doubt (my initial defensive startle) may give way to patience amid awe (an opening of the mind via expansion of inner space) as the path toward the deeper reaches of reality.

Mindfulness and the implicate order (Bohm): recognising the animate and inanimate as two phases of a unified reality

This expansion of mental and emotional space, accompanied by awe, is often considered in terms of mindfulness. We have seen from a neuro-scientific view (Solms, 2013), that there is a neural network that monitors the external world, which links us with memory and cognition, and an internal network that attends to our inner self-regulatory functions, and registers our sense of well-being via affect. Usually, the brain can focus on only one network at a time, but studies (Jospiovic et al., 2012; Ricard, et al., 2014) have shown that those who are very familiar with meditation can maintain both networks' activity simultaneously. This dual activity leads to mediation of intense affect without being swept away.

> . . . (N)euroscience research has shown that *experienced meditators could keep both networks active at the same time while they meditated. Doing so lowered the wall between the self and environment, possibly with the effect of inspiring feelings of harmony with the world.* This ability is called *non-duality,* or oneness in both Eastern and Western philosophies [Jospiovic, Z., Denstein, I., Weber, J., & Heeger, D.J. (2012). The influence of meditation on anti-correlated networks in the brain. *Frontiers in Human Neuroscience, 5*: 1–11] (as quoted in Nichols, 2014, pp. 232–233, my emphasis)]

Specifically, meditators in studies with control groups demonstrate more capacity to experience raw affects and pain than non-meditator controls. They are less overwhelmed by their own and others' pain and are able to feel more positive emotions related to compassion, rather than negative emotions related to burnout by the distress. The research suggests that meditators have been able to sustain

> the coordination of brain oscillations [which] . . . may play a potentially crucial role in the brain's building of temporary networks that

can *integrate cognitive and affective functions during learning and conscious perception, a process that can bring about lasting changes in brain circuitry.* (Ricard et al., 2014, p. 45, my emphasis)

These brain oscillations would probably equate with Solms' description of cognitive cortical functions binding or transforming the affect or free energy (my defensive response to my patient's intense complaint) into a representation (the image of the islands), which binds the affect. In the first-person subjective experience, and from EEG evidence, meditators experience the usually stable sense of self as becoming less fixed and permanent, probably because the sense of harmony and flow offers a more containing representation, binding free energy (anxiety) and reducing the need for certainty as to "who we are" and "what we know". The more harmonious sense of unity probably decreases the terrors of uncertainty and, thus, also the defensive need for absolute and concrete experience.

From another viewpoint, McGilchrist (2009, p. 207) suggests that the annihilation of the self in Buddhist tradition might be the dissolving of the boundary of one's individuality by pouring oneself out into a larger vessel, as it were. As bud into flower into fruit (*Aufhebogen*), one is transformed or mingled into the more complex manifestations of an ultimate unity.

Similarly, David Bohm (1980,1996), a physicist well versed in eastern and western views of the nature of reality, suggests that the universe might usefully be regarded as a continuous field in flux. He says that our human ways of viewing it, which inevitably involve differentiation and parsing that unity, present a view of reality as fragmented into "this" and "that", "these" and "those", "us" and "them", which can then lead to a more fixed, and absolute sense of "what is". Bohm (1980) suggests that the deepest, widest, most unified reality is one of constant motion involving both implicate (enfolded) and explicate (unfolded) elements in constant fluctuation, so that what is in the background and implicit one moment becomes foreground and explicit the next (1980, pp. 258–260.)

Bohm, then, is suggesting that both the conscious explicit experience and the unconscious implicit elements are phases of the same unitary reality. To my mind this description aligns with the experience of the meditators, as well as to my emerging imagery in the last vignette of the several islands surrounded by a connecting sea.

He suggests that we can pay attention in a way to overcome our necessary fragmentation of reality: sustained enquiry into the exercise of attention and recognition of our assumptions as just that—as assumptions rather than truths—aids in the recognition of the "fragmentation of the world . . . which arises from our need for our language-rooted . . . thought processes" (Bohm, 1996, p. xxvii). Such recognition would allow one to come closer to the implicate order, the unfolding and enfolding of deeper reality, closer to "O", in Bion's terms.

Bohm feels that we learn to pay attention to the explicit order, in terms of our daily life and activities. But, he says, we also need to pay attention increasingly to the implicit, the "unlimited", in his phrase. This best occurs when we shift our attention from the details and the noise of everyday life, he suggests, which, by definition, is explicit in its limitations and fantasy of control. Focus on the implicit really occurs in quiet calm space, where, in the lack of focus, one can attend to the emerging subtleties of the implicit, that wider aspect of being, and flow and harmony (1996, pp.106–108). This quality of attention offers "a relaxed, non-judgmental curiosity, its primary activity being to see things as freshly and clearly as possible" (Bohm, 1996, p. xviii). How interesting that non-judgemental curiosity is also what is described as the poetic stance in our review of poetry. And it may be the process one engages in with at-one-ment, which is Bion's notion of being.

This open dialogic process amid quietude, allowing fresh, emerging views, might well be what also occurs internally within the individual during meditation, when there is simultaneous attention to one's cognitive and affective functions. This view might also be illustrated by my own experience of widening the field as I experienced my patient's intense complaint. My first (affective) impulse was defensive, but that was mediated by my awareness that I needed to remain non-reactive and to seek a larger container. I believe my doing so was employing non-judgemental curiosity to view not only my patient's intensely experienced concern, but also the awareness of the different context I held toward "the problem". The resulting image, several islands and their surrounding sea, served as a fresh, clear view of the current situation, rather than as a pressured chamber where one intense complaint dominated the space.

Bohm's term for this quality of thought so prominent in genuine dialogue is "participatory thought" (1996, pp. 96–109), a type of thought where boundaries are softened, and are felt to be permeable, along with a sense of an underlying relatedness among all the participants. From this view, absolute categories recede in meaning, as does the clear demarcation between animate and inanimate. This recession of categories is exemplified by Bohm's wondering whether minerals essential for living organisms, such as sodium, calcium, and potassium, are inanimate or animate when they are part of living systems. He suggests, then, that the ongoing flux between the animate and the inanimate is best considered as two phases of a unified reality.

Bion's vertex of at-one-ment might be very similar (Sandler, 2005, pp. 60–65). He suggests that explicit experience includes registrations of material reality, which can be put into words. Psychic reality, however, that which is implicit, in the same way Bohm describes, cannot be put into words. It can only be opened up to and lived. In my vignette, my refraining from reactivity and opening my view to the wider reality (as represented by the image of several islands and their surrounding sea) could be viewed as a moment of at-one-ment, because I had faith that such an opening would deepen the possible realisations which could only be intuited. According to Sandler (2005) *at-one-ment* ". . . describe[s] situations that are experientially alive and truthful . . . formulat[ing] an evolving ultimate reality during the here and now". . . . It is not a tool to *know* psychic reality, but to *apprehend* it in a transient way" (p. 60). I believe that is what occurred in the vignette once I could open up past my momentary reactivity.

All of these viewpoints suggest that coming alive involves submitting hard-edged thought to the softer sense of intuition. That is, opening up mental space involves the softening of edges, while remaining hardened closes down and strangles the rhythms needed for transformation. The propaganda of the left-hemispheric functions then, offering language, detail, and precision, promises certainty as *the* way forward. This allure might actually be an agent for the ego's yearning toward sleep, as Solms warns us. The biologic pressures toward automaticity add to those tendencies of the left-hemispheric functions. Articulating that voice of the left hemisphere, I would say:

> It is too hard, too frustrating, too much work to stay open, alive, questing, uncertain. Let me rest on my laurels, keep my tenure, remain loyal to my theory and my secure identity. Let me stay invested in my greed and exploitation and thus remain indifferent to its effects upon the living,

breathing planet. Let me stay invested in my certainty and thus hallucinated power, which means having no openness to widening perspectives,
nor to exploration of the new and as yet undiscovered, implicit aspects of
reality.

The legacy of the fall from certainty, viewed as the idealised bliss
of remaining undisturbed by change, may be seen as the hard work of
coming alive, awakening, swimming against the biological pressure
toward automaticity. This may be part of becoming.

Heidegger: being (Dasein) and care (Sorge)

These considerations about coming alive might, in part, be the legacy
of the philosophical trends in the twentieth century that demonstrate
this shift from cognitive knowing about reality in a declarative, definitive fashion towards the realisation that reality is more complex than
human capacities can fully comprehend, and is, thus, best approached
via lived experience.

Martin Heidegger may be considered to epitomise this view. In *Sein
und Zeit* (1927) (*Being and Time*, 1996), considered by many to be his
pinnacle work, Heidegger suggests a hidden, ever-evolving reality
that he notes as *Sein* (Being.) It can be engaged by human capacities in
a limited fashion by way of a patient, attentive process of being-in-the-
world, which Heidegger terms *Dasein*. For Heidegger, *Dasein* involves
a fulsome engagement of the everyday senses moment by moment, in
a wide-ranging, receptive way. Here, the individual adopts a stance
of humility, rather than of declaration and certainty, one of patient
responsiveness to the as yet undisclosed aspects of implicit reality.
Steiner (1978) describes Heidegger's view as man's being "a privileged
listener and respondent to existence . . . [of] trying 'to listen to the voice
of Being'" (pp. 29–31). These views about approaching reality seem to
be very consonant with those of Bion and Bohm.

Appreciating the implicit suggests also being open to metaphor,
that is, viewing beyond the surface toward depth and context. Heidegger might say that we need to listen to what emerges from our
language rather than to close the space by quickly imposing ideas
upon that language. But he might also agree that, at times, we need to
understand in a linear way, as do the left-brain functions, before we

can engage with, or, rather, allow the metaphoric potential of the right to emerge and to enrich our experience in terms of glimpsing of, rather than grasping at, reality. Heidegger also suggests that if we can listen to the Being within ourselves with the same open-hearted responsiveness, we may witness, even foster, the emergence of our own hidden creativity.

The embracing ambience for this reciprocal engagement at all levels is one of wide-ranging care and concern (*Sorge*). For Heidegger *Sorge* is fundamental to our way of being (*Dasein*) (Ladson Hinton, 17 November 2015 (personal communication)), a concept being revealed in the chapters of this book. Heidegger's view of a unified reality, approached more by lived rather than cognitively based experience, almost precisely aligns with the views put forth by Bohm and the later works of Bion. That his writing preceded these other authors by a few decades further underscores his influence in twentieth century thinking, not only in philosophy but also in other branches of the humanities and psychology. The convergence of these authors' thoughts about faith in one's intuitive experience over the efforts of cognition to grasp and posses truth and reality further affirms the value of lived experience.

CHAPTER SEVEN

Being: remaining open to learn from evolving experience. A personal exploration

I n efforts to learn from life's experiences, the paradox of wishing to grow but also wishing not to be disturbed is encountered. There is the wish to flourish, but also the wish to avoid the disturbance that inevitably accompanies that growth.

A note from my own experience might exemplify this human dilemma. After years in the field of psychoanalysis, while savouring the many opportunities to learn in a relaxed open-ended way, I was also encountering the more fatiguing tensions which are endemic when one privileges certain ways of thinking, and certain schools of thought. While theories are important as scaffoldings for learning and as ways to structure experience, they also parse the flow of experience, as does language. And when one is confronted in the moment with intense unmediated affect, whether one's own anxiety, or the complexity of the implicit–explicit flow of emotion, whether within the self or between individuals, it is tempting to freeze the frame, to label and categorise in order to quell the anxiety and perhaps even the terror one may feel in the moment. It is very difficult to remain unknowing amid the tensions of clinical work.

Even more complex are the pulls towards enactment. Most clinicians accept the fact that we resort to enactment until we can think about the pressures that fuel the action. Enactments, like dreams, may be implicit communications about what cannot yet be explicitly known. None the less, psychoanalytic education usually urges that enactments be subjected to understanding (thoughts instead of action) as soon as possible, out of respect for the underlying forces considered as impulses (or unmediated affects), which might foster traumatic repetitions rather than creative engagements. Again, important reasons to invoke thoughtful transformations.

As a student of medicine in the 1960s, I was taught repeatedly about the need for careful, even precise observation along with the wider-ranging diagnostic thinking about what these observations might indicate. These lessons expanded the acuity and agility of my mind, but alongside was the rather constant pressure to "get it right" and to do so "as quickly as possible", which made it very difficult to allow a relaxed curiosity to come into play. This manner of learning and exploration under pressure, useful in many medical situations requiring rapid responses to protect life and limb, also enhanced for me the narcissistic vulnerability that "not getting it right the first time" could lead to the dread of failure and humiliation.

Psychoanalytic training and practice has offered the opportunity to unlearn some of those hard-edged lessons of medical training, but the theories taught as scaffolds for organising the flow of experience also serve necessarily to parse reality. Ways to categorise certain psychic phenomena, such as "transference" or "resistance", aids in organising, but also inevitably contributes to freezing the frame. This is similar to the mother's label "yellow" for the patch of sunshine on the nursery wall, closing down the child's wonder about the sun.

Theories, then, offer ways to organise the data, crucial in one's early learning. However, they are only guidelines to follow, not to be idealised or concretised as *the* definitions of reality. Still, I fear that, subject to Solm's observation, the ego wants to submit to automaticity and it is tugged by the tendency to concretise and to idealise. These tendencies freeze the frame and surrender any questing amid uncertainty. Theories, which become "realities", or unquestioned authorities, are examples of such. Idealising a theory or a mentor sidesteps personal navigation by projecting one's own authority outward, more or less saying "he knows the way, he will lead me into certainty". Idealisation recreates the stance of Chuster's medieval Christian man, or simulates reversion to the all-providing womb that promises the blissful paradise of certainty from pain and doubt.

Still, the invitation to lean on another's authority is very powerful: developing a school of thought might initially be the creative exploration of new territory. But, over time, institutional elements set in and the freshness and intimate explorations give way to "standards" and doctrinal thought. This automatising pattern seems endemic in academic and religious history and, perhaps, states of fatigue and stasis in any field.

Several years ago, after decades of study in my field, I began to feel saturated by inevitable tendencies towards tribal loyalties regarding schools of thought and hierarchies where ideas were presented as psychic truths. Trained in the USA and in London, I was influenced by Freudian, Kleinian, and Bionian thought. While I had for years manifestly supported pluralism, learning from each other psychoanalytically, I had begun to feel that I was in the middle of inevitable tribal wranglings as to who was closest to the psychoanalytic "truth". Perhaps due to institutional forces, while amid earnest minds trying to learn, I felt an ancient pressure to conform or to idealise. This actually partially closed my mind to open efforts and explorations. This is an example of the gravitational pull toward concretisation and automaticity. The sense of hardening edges, and urges to accept this truth over that one, fatigued my ability to softly learn amid relaxed curiosity, that is, to follow Bohm's description of transforming dialogue.

In an effort to rescue and to open my partially closed mind, I decided to seek other avenues of learning. For some time, I had been interested in the nature of reality, the common ground behind the many divergent views about the topic from thoughtful perspectives. Perhaps, like Poggio (Greenblatt, 2011), in search of ancient wisdom (*De rerum natura*) about the Epicurean sentiments savouring lived experience, I sought sources outside my field, antidotes, I hoped, to my beleaguered state of mind. Looking back, I might have been searching intuitively for ways to come alive, to regain that creative dialogic stance internally or with colleagues. With a little online research, I had the good fortune to contact someone who has pursued a dual track interest for decades: astrophysics and contemplations about being. I visited Piet Hut, Chair of Interdisciplinary Studies at his office at the Institute for Advanced Studies at Princeton, in 2008, mentioning that I was interested in reaching beyond my field of psychoanalysis, while utilising its insights when applicable, to further explore the nature of reality. He said he was about to begin an online forum for dialogic explorations on the nature of being which might enhance my quest. Did I wish to join that effort? Indeed I did.

These explorations, involving a new medium for me, the virtual world, were quite intense at times. A significant community varying in membership, background, and experience continued for the several years of my active participation, and a smaller community still continues its daily explorations in the same venue. Professor Hut's hope was to establish a community that fostered dialogue about the nature of being, as part of the nature of reality. For me, the being that Piet suggests is similar to what Bion terms as "O", the ultimate, unfathomable reality. Piet's overview and summation of his experience during that project are taken from a recent online interview (Hut, 2014).

Regarding the task at hand, given our manner of parsing reality, Piet says,

> Being cannot be defined, because any definition delineates what something is in contrast to what it is not. Given that Being's nature is what is, in the widest sense of the word, it cannot be contrasted to anything else. If you want to try to be logical about it, you could say: Being points beyond existence and non-existence, beyond what is and is not in our normal use of the word . . .

In order to begin to explore being, he says,

> What we would need is a dialogue in which two or more people engage in a conversation in which they walk around the topic, weaving more and more context in which slowly more and more of the contours of our way of dealing with the notion of Being are outlined to at least some extent. Being itself can not be outlined, because it does not have a contour or edge or limit; but our ways of dealing with Being can.

> And this is not so strange. Language uses words and concepts that act as filters or fisherman's nets. Each word means this and not that, points at one class of things or actions as opposed to another one. Being as a word that point(s) to the ultimate "what IS" simply cannot be caught in a net, we cannot fish for Being. Being is as much fish as water as net as fisherman, [it] can't be divided.

Dialogue, once again, as a way to explore approaches to being:

> the only way Being can take on more meaning for a . . . community, is to have a sustained community conversation . . . [and] for such a conversation to be alive and meaningful . . . [it is important that] each member of that . . . community . . . [draw upon] . . . [his/her] own life as a laboratory, rather than drawing mostly upon outside authorities . . . (Hut, 2014)

Piet fostered that community conversation in the online explorations. Having meeting times throughout the day to accommodate participants via their avatars from all over the world in online discussion, he established a scaffolding to hold and to gather the group. His dedication and leadership were gifts to all who came, whether for a time or two or for more ongoing participation. His patience and generosity in conveying his understandings about being, and "playing as being", as the project came to be called, were gifts to us all. He truly wished to aid others in attaining the unity of mind that he and other meditators had done over a period of many years. Part of his wish was that those many years of contemplations could be shortened and played out within the "play as being" community. I was part of that community for several years, learning as I could, offering psychoanalytic understandings as applicable. All of us grew in our capacities for openness and awe, broadening our perspectives, and deepening our insights. Piet had the foresight to arrange for an online archive from which these quotations about his vision are taken. (https://wiki. playasbeing.org/chronicles/the_chapter_31:_pema_pera_interview.)

He also felt that the deeper dialogues about being that he notes as so important in these explorations did not take root as deeply as he had wished. He wonders whether these contemplations were just too alien or alienating for most participants. Looking back at my experience, a few thoughts about the "why" come to mind. I think that Piet's charismatic presence, and his significant base of knowledge and experience in meditation and in other ways, automatically made him an authority in our eyes. I think I did not realise how great that influence was at the time. In discussions, including reading some of the sources that had inspired him, the community continued to privilege his efforts on our behalf rather than our own often nascent experience. His considerable efforts to get us to use our own "life as a lab", that is, relying on our own experience rather than the authority of others, were very helpful, but still, they could not restrain our idealisation of him.

There was also the sense of the concept of being as probably too alien to be able to grapple with outside of his tutelage. We all might have minimised the tendency to rely on his authority in these matters.

As well, at least for me, the online experience, while exciting and visually spectacular, invited complete immersion. Yet, as such, it also became a bubble experience to some extent. It was difficult for me to fully internalise the alluring environment as part of my own authentic, ongoing self. Perhaps more experience in the virtual world would have been helpful for me in this regard.

I offer this possibility, familiarity with context, because I have had an in person experience which I think approximated the depth of dialogue Piet had hoped could be sustained. The format was small group meetings with the same group of eight to ten people for a few set hours a day over several days in a lovely setting, where all the group members engaged in listening and commenting on each other's clinical work. What enhanced the dialogic experience, in my view, was the nature of the leadership. While there was an agenda, listening to each other's cases with an eye on learning, the titular leader, someone who had organised the meeting and the housekeeping issues, was a person who also set the tone of complete egalitarianism. He modelled in manner and tone that we were all on a level playing field. In a very subtle and perhaps not entirely conscious way, he conveyed that he did not have anything special to teach; he was present entirely as a co-participant, eager to learn with and from us all. Within this atmosphere, some extraordinary things occurred: with no defined authority but still a definite task, a sense of mutual trust and respect soon developed. Within that atmosphere we could all listen, and be moved and respond from emotional and intuitive, rather than intellectual, sources. It felt that the contributions from all participants, from the very young in age and experience to the older members of the group, were sensitive, intuitive, and seemed to emerge from emotional experience rather than theoretical considerations. This became the basis of our work together. That atmosphere of trust and sharing felt deeply moving for each and all.

This experience altered my view of learning from an authorised consultant, helping me to realise how the presence of an authority automatically triggers that sense of hierarchical structure within the group, and, indeed, within the individual. This could be important when basic learning is required, such as in medical training, or any basic learning of a set of skills and procedures. However, having a designated authority stands in contrast to the genuine dialogic learning which I now feel can occur only amid trust and a non-authoritarian atmosphere. One could consider that left hemispheric functions come into predominance when authority is on the scene. By this, I mean that one feels invited, perhaps out of ancestral pressures towards tribal authority, to idealise the authoritative other and his productions and to devalue one's own quieter perceptions or emerging intuitions. Indeed, this pressure to idealise authority was the mind-closing situation, which had triggered my explorations beyond my field in the first place.

I believe this is the kind of experience Piet Hut had hoped for in the online explorations.

Finally, regarding the ongoing question about the nature of reality, Piet offers the following thoughts:

> What is the nature of reality? Or, to unpack that a bit more: what is the world like, that it offers so many different perspectives to different individuals, or even to the same individual at different times? . . . I see humanity's homework for the twenty-first century, and beyond, as starting to integrate the piecemeal answers that have been obtained, winnowing out what is more universal from the more tribal parts of the answers so far. Whether such a more and more enlarged view of reality will be called science or philosophy or by other names is less important than the fact that it is high time to start this kind of global effort . . . (Hut, 2014)

Perhaps this book's explorations provide some glimpses about a wider reality that seems to consist of flows of energy. Human perspectives arise from capacities to differentiate from that (in our eyes) "inanimate" energy field. Our development parses reality into various digestible chunks, by way of distinctions, separations, sequences, and symbols. The evolutionary legacy of affective upwelling energises and terrifies us. Cortical processes, derived from experience and memory, such as those of maternal care, attempt to shape and to gentle that upwelling in ways that foster perceptions and growing senses about ourselves. Part of that management is the development of language, which aids in thinking about, and manipulation of, ourselves and the world. Biologically, this sophisticated way of viewing ourselves is vastly expensive of energy, inviting us to relegate all learning to automatic functions, and then to turn away from the pain of staying alive and of appreciating the beauty of the world.

The cost of this differentiation is that we lose touch with the wider realities, the cosmos both internal and external, which might help us to keep things in perspective. To see ourselves as small and in awe would aid healthy appreciation of our true place in either realm, but our intellectual powers, perhaps in part fuelled by the forces unleashed by the upwelling, often convince us that we are in charge of the universe, a dangerous position to assume. This hubris might dovetail with mythic tendencies to imagine a Paradise, where there is no separation from the all-powerful source of life, be it God, or the mother and her body. The allure for that return, ironically, is probably part of the invitation for the ego's slumber. It takes energy, pain, and the tolerance of doubt to leave that Garden, to venture into uncertainty, and to grow. The question is, how to retain awe and wonder, those links that foster the growth of inner space, as reliable portals toward deepening appreciation of reality.

The innate preconception of care as the affirmation of being

One thing that seems central in our musings is the expectation of maternal care. Mammalian evolution has probably hard-wired this anticipation of warmth and care into mediating the processes that foster coming alive. When this prediction is met, one feels affirmed and seen, inner space is engaged, and one experiences a deepening sense of enlivenment. When the preconception of care is *not* met, there is no Garden of well-being to offer a base of nourishment and growth. Instead, one feels closer to being cast adrift in a terrifying universe fuelled by unmediated affect, which might be experienced as intense pressure or as cruel and castigating internal voices. Care, concern, and engagement, which mediate the terror of untamed affect, are essential to coming alive and sustaining our becoming and our being.

Still, once the thinking self is engaged, there is a natural resistance to open oneself to that preconception. That is, to trust in that care anticipated but not yet manifest. Because to do so means to turn away from the fantasied safety of intellectual distance, in order to once again allow oneself into the sweep of experience, with no guarantees of fulfilment. As we have seen, that immersion in itself does not offer the illusion of control and mastery. In fact, the intellectual self declares that it is foolish to give up the security of clear thought, to throw away a sure thing in order to trust in dreams or shadows. In these circumstances, it takes faith to privilege the wider, deeper potential of our intuition, that internalised residence of care, concern, and engagement. *Faith, in this circumstance, might simply be trusting more in our intuition than in our intellect,* and that faith might be sorely tested by the allure of the intellect and the unsettling of doubt.

This predominance of our intellect and our fear of our unmediated affect might be why we do not seem to manage becoming and being very well. We tend to be swept into obsessive thought or violent action, rather than to rest in quiet curiosity. We might be at the cusp, however, if we can harness our omnipotence and if we can recognise the value, as well as the limitations, of our left-hemispheric thought. These efforts allow us to appreciate the quiet contemplations that allow us to reconnect with our right-hemispheric intuitions. If we can realise that the explicit and implicit aspects of experience are all part of one reality, such as by engaging in transformative dialogue, rather than seeking one authority, if we can remain humble in the face of the wider, deeper reality, and if we can surrender the products of our significant mental achievements to these quieter, more humble intuitive roots, then we might be more in awe and less in dread. Privileging the receptive, intuitive aspects of the right hemisphere invokes the process of *being* rather than *thinking about* reality.

Again, it might be that faith in our intuition rather than our intellect is key to this transformation.

*   *   *

Are these musings in themselves explorations into the nature of reality? Are they glimpses of the wider reality beyond our usual view? Are they versions of "from bud to flower to fruit" transformations? Is the capacity for evolution, whether of the cosmos, or the plant, or the human individual part of the nature of reality? This book's various explorations into the processive nature of reality would suggest that this is so. However, being creatures of evolution, we might not be able to envision a reality without this flow. Such would be too foreign, perhaps, envisioning too vacant a world, or a universe without recognisable life. The nature of reality, then, for us, may embrace the ongoing processes "becoming and "being". That is, the quiet explorations of ever-emerging emotional understandings.

CHAPTER EIGHT

Epigenetics: the impact of immediate experience upon our genes might demonstrate the power as well as the wisdom of lived experience

I would like to end with a few words about the impact of immediate experience. This last chapter, a coda of sorts, glances at the power of lived experience in terms we are just beginning to understand. Epigenetics is informing us that our everyday experience has a rather immediate impact on genetic expression. While there is still debate amid the epigenetic community about what conclusions can be drawn from these observations, it appears that this burgeoning field is demonstrating that gene expression might be influenced profoundly by our often rather immediate experience. Dobbs (2013), Weinhold (2006), and Laland and colleagues (2014), summarising significant epigenetic research, suggest that experience might alter our cellular function almost immediately, not by changing the DNA sequencing of genes, but by altering gene expression. It seems that even moment-by-moment experience directly impacts how much or how little certain genes express themselves. For instance, genetically gentle bees placed in the same environment with aggressive bees become more and more aggressive, due to altered gene expression. As well, aggressive Africanised bees become gentled when raised in the hives of less aggressive bees. Being in the same environment triggers genetic switches so that, in this instance, the bees become increasingly like their hive-mates, not only behaviourally, but also genetically. Close examination reveals that their gene expression has been changed often within minutes or hours, by experience, probably an evolutionary advantage for survival in changing circumstances.

In a small freshwater fish, the African cichlid, it has been observed that only one male can be dominant in any given population at any one time. One epigenetic investigator and his team (Chen & Fernald, 2006) were astonished to see that if the dominant male is removed, the next in the hierarchy within minutes will adopt the flashy colours and activity level that only the dominant male displays. Before the observers' eyes the number two fish becomes number one, even increasing in size to accommodate his new status, thanks entirely to the change of environment, that is, either the suppression of genetic expression in the presence of the former dominant male, or the excitation of certain dominance characteristics due to the previous rival's absence. This is a dramatic example of one's environment rapidly shaping gene expression and one's whole way of being.

Epigeneticists, observing the human susceptibility to illness across several populations, find similar patterns of gene expression in those described as feeling socially insecure or alone (Cole, 2009). What the epigeneticist might call social isolation, or loneliness (Cacioppo & Patrick, 2008) the psychologist or psychoanalyst might view as a vulnerable sense of self, or the internalisation of a depressed or absent caring object. In any event, the experience of the lack of care or accompaniment seems to heighten our susceptibility to illness via gene suppression of the immune system. It has also been observed (Kaufman et al., 2004) that the presence of one reliable caring person can make all the difference for a vulnerable individual in terms of recovery of the immune system. It is interesting to consider whether the wider picture here is that there are various physical and emotional manifestations of inadequate protection: at the emotional level, feelings of isolation and of vulnerability and even of terror; at the physiological and cellular level, weakened resilience of the immune system.

If we are essentially social beings, then, there is very probably an innate expectation of social inclusion, which, when met, registers the sense of well-being in the face of (and resilience against) the internal and external forces which could destabilise that well-being. It might be that several bodily processes respond in concert when the basic expectation of care and belonging is *not* experienced. Neurologically, the free energy, uncontained by cortical processes (attentive care gone awry), disrupts; immunologically, there is less resilience in the immune system. That is, less capacity to protect against over-inflammation in its combat against internal or external threats to the body. Psychologically, we have been used to considering despair in terms of depression, the predominance of a deadened internal object, or somehow the psyche turning away from life. We might, in short, be viewing several manifestations of the same phenomenon: the preconception of care, accompaniment, and social engagement, the default state for human beings, being unmet.

We have known psychologically and, more recently, neurologically, how such care impacts human development. It is interesting now to see that such experience also becomes etched in our cells. Good care apparently leaves its mark in cell memory. And the absence of such care, or the presence of trauma and neglect, also, we assume, leaves a mark. Our subjective experience is carried in our cells as a consequence of immediate experience, but also as a legacy for our personal future, and perhaps that of our children and their children as well. With these accruing understandings, one wonders anew about the impact of war zones and continuing trauma for children who have spent years in such environments. The literature from this perspective might be accruing.

We have generally thought of ourselves as distinct individuals passing through the world we live in. But

> ... what we're learning from the molecular processes that actually keep our bodies running is that we're far more fluid than we realise, and the world passes through us which changes us, often nearly on the spot to adapt to the immediate environment. (Dobbs, 2013)

"This is what a cell is about", epigenetics expert John Cole says. "A cell ... is a machine for turning experience into biology" (Dobbs, 2013).

"The world passes through us" offers the perspective of our transience, our susceptibility to the influence of experience, our being imprinted by the forces around us—perhaps restoring the sense of our smallness in terms of the universe. For example, we are only beginning to understand how much we are impacted not only physically but emotionally by the micro-organisms which inhabit in our intestinal tract (Schmidt, 2015). The mutual influence between our emotional selves and that biome is only beginning to be understood.

In addition, "a cell . . . is a machine for turning experience into biology" offers the sense of how mutable we are, not at all the crisply defined individuals separate from the flow of being that we might imagine. We might also be warned, however, that the metaphor of cell-as-machine hints at how we may simultaneously view these sites of physical transformation (cellular processes) in mechanical terms. Quite simply, we do not as yet have the vocabulary to view these intricate systems that bind our experience into our biological makeup. We barely know how to think about them. Perhaps we can develop more descriptive terms and concepts as we better understand these bodily imprints of our experience, while also keeping an eye on the left hemisphere's ever-present tendency to mechanise (cell as machine) what might be some of the most exquisite and yet potent notations and expressions of our lived experience.

*   *   *

Here, then, is more tangible evidence of the impact of lived experience, which brings us full circle back to Poggio's search for ancient wisdom, the Epicurean sentiments expressed by Lucretius in *De rerum Natura* (The Nature of Things). We might better appreciate how the mind-closing nature of authority, whether Rome, the Church, or our internal de-animating urges, may be gently opposed by our embodied experience. That is, embodied experience that gives rise to our intuitions as well as the more robust genetic expressions that shape our immediate and more distant future. The power as well as the wisdom of lived experience may be dawning upon our awareness.

NOTES

1. In his substantial work *The Language of Bion* (2005) Paulo Sandler, in the entry on "Become, Becoming" writes,

   Analysis is a practical, living experience . . . In order to emphasize this with its built-in, ever-changing nature, Bion resorts to the term, "becoming". In *A Memoir of the Future*, there are three ficti- tious characters . . . who may be seen as steps towards becoming who one is . . . All of them correspond to Bion's memories of his own learning from experience . . . reflecting his own trajectory in life . . . There are many parts of the text (Memoire) that offer opportunities to see the integration and the disintegration of a whole life, being lived in a moment—the moment one "becomes". Life, after all, only exists in the moment it is being lived . . . Becoming may be seen as a continuous process during a life cycle . . . It is becoming who one is in reality. (pp. 75–76)

2. Quoting Frances Tustin, and Daniel Stern, Ogden mentions how difficult it is to articulate these shapes into words because of their pre-symbolic nature. He suggests that the intermediate space between these modes, or poles, of experience is the locus of experience, and that collapse towards any pole can occur.

> Collapse toward the autistic–contiguous pole generates imprison-
> ment in the machine-like tyranny of attempted sensory-based
> escape from the terror of formless dread by means of reliance on
> rigid defenses. Collapse into the paranoid–schizoid pole is charac-
> terized by imprisonment in a non-subjective world of thoughts
> and feelings experienced in terms of frightening and protective
> things that simply happen and cannot be thought about or inter-
> preted. Collapse in the direction of the depressive pole involves a
> form of isolation of oneself from one's bodily sensations and from
> the immediacy of one's lived experience leaving one devoid of
> spontaneity and aliveness . . . (1998, p. 42)

3. The concept of splitting will be revisited from a neuroscientific view (see
    Chapter Two) in terms of the interference with the right posterior hemi-
    sphere's capacities to establish external and internal space.

4. This is close to the position of Allan Schore (2011), who states that the
    cleavage of implicit experience as seen in dissociation and disavowal
    precedes and dominates over repression as a psychic organiser.

5. This very collapse of "lived experience" is described by Solms' detailed
    view of the functions of the right perisylvan region, as viewed through
    lesion studies, which provides more compelling evidence about the right
    hemisphere as the seat of the vitalising, or animating, functions.

6. The opening meditation of Chapter Four describes the interface between
    these two ways of being.

7. The confabulation "My brother's arm" can be described from varying
    views: earlier, Solms suggests it as a primitive defence against the
    unbearable pain which accompanies the reversion to the narcissistic point
    of view about disability; here, McGilchrist's views about the confabula-
    tory nature of the unmediated left hemisphere is cited. Multiple views,
    allowing a flexible rather than a narrowing single perspective, foster a
    rounded picture of the complexity of psychic functioning.

8. See beginning of Chapter Five for an illustration of the experience at this
    interface.

REFERENCES

Anderson, M. (1999). The pressure toward enactment and the hatred of reality. *Journal of the American Psychoanalytic Association, 47*: 503–518.

Andrade, V. M. (2005). Affect and the therapeutic action of psychoanalysis. *International Journal of Psychoanalysis, 86*: 677–697.

Andrade, V. M. (2007). Dreaming as a primordial state of the mind: the clinical relevance of structural faults in the body ego as revealed in dreaming. *International Journal of Psychoanalysis, 88*: 55–74.

Anzieu, D. (1986). Paradoxical transference: from paradoxical communication to negative therapeutic reaction. *Contemporary Psychoanalysis, 22*: 520–547.

Ariely, D. (2008). Why do placebos work? https://www.youtube.com/watch?v=bHBwHVbUwig (accessed on 3 November 2015).

Bass, A. (1997). The problem of "concreteness". *Psychoanalytic Quarterly, 66*: 642–682.

Bass, A. (2000). *Difference and Disavowal: The Trauma of Eros*. Palo Alto, CA: Stanford University Press.

Berlin, H. A. (2011). The neural basis of the dynamic unconscious. *Neuropsychoanalysis, 13*: 5–31.

Bion, W. R. (1957). The differentiation of the psychotic from the non-psychotic personality. *International Journal of Psychoanalysis, 38*: 266–275.

Bion, W. R. (1965). *Transformations: Change from Learning to Growth*. Bath: Pitman Press.

Bion, W. R. (1967). *Second Thoughts*. London: Heinemann Medical Books.

Bion, W. R. (1970). *Attention and Interpretation: A Scientific Approach to Insight in Psycho-analysis and Groups*. London: Tavistock.

Blass, R. (2014). On 'the fear of death' as the primary anxiety: how and why Klein differs from Freud. *International Journal of Psychoanalysis, 95*: 613–627.

Blass, R. B. (2015). Conceptualizing splitting: on the different meanings of splitting and their implications for the understanding of the person and the analytic process, *International Journal of Psychoanalysis, 96*: 123–139.

Bohm, D. (1980). *Wholeness and the Implicate Order*. London: Routledge [reprinted 1992].

Bohm, D. (1996). *On Dialogue*. London: Routledge.

Bolte Taylor, J. (2008a). *My Stroke of Insight*. London: Hodder & Stoughton.

Bolte Taylor, J. (2008b). Jill bolte Taylor's stroke of insight. February. TED podcast. www.ted.com;talks'jill_bolte_taylor_s_powerful_stroke_of_insight.html (accessed on 3 November 2015).

Botella, C. (2014). On remembering: the notion of memory without recollection. *International Journal of Psychoanalysis, 95*: 911–936.

Cacioppo, J. & Patrick, W. (2009). *Loneliness: Human Nature and the Need for Social Connection*. New York: Norton.

Carhart-Harris, R., & Friston, K. (2010). The default-mode, ego functions and free energy: a neurobiological account of Freudian ideas. *Brain, 133*(4): 1265–1283.

Chen, C. C., & Fernald, R. D. (2006). Distributions of two gonadotropin-releasing hormone receptor types in a cichlid fish suggest functional specialization. *Journal of Comparative Neurology, 495*(3): 314–323.

Chuster, A. (2014). The myth of Satan. In: *A Lonesome Road: Essays on the Complexity of W. R. Bion's Work*. Trio Studio Grafica Digital, www.triostudio.com.br (accessed 3 November 2015).

Cimino, C., & Correale, A. (2005). Projective identification and consciousness alteration: a bridge between psychoanalysis and neuroscience? *International Journal of Psychoanalysis, 86*: 51–60.

Civitarese, G. (2013). *The Violence of Emotions: Bion and Post-Bionian Psychoanalysis*. London: Routledge.

Civitarese, G. (2014). Bion and the sublime: the origins of an aesthetic paradigm. *International Journal of Psychoanalysis, 95*: 1059–1086.

Civitarese, G. (2015). Transformations in hallucinosis and the receptivity of the analyst. *International Journal of Psychoanalysis, 96*(4): 1091–1116.

Cole, S. (2009). Social regulation of human gene expression. *Current Directions in Psychological Science, 18*(3): 132–137.

Crick, F., & Mitchison, G. (1983). The function of dream sleep. *Nature, 304*(5922): 111–114.

Damasio, A. (2010). *Self Comes to Mind*. New York: Pantheon.

Diamond, M. (In press). The return of the "Repressed": dissociation and the psychoanalysis of the traumatized mind. In: T. McBride & M. Murphy (Eds.), *Trauma, Destruction and Transformative Potential*. London: Karnac.

Divino, C. L., & Moore, M. S. (2010). Integrating neurobiological findings into psychodynamic psychotherapy training and practice. *Psychoanalytic Dialogues, 20*: 337–355.

Dobbs, D. (2013). The social life of genes. *Pacific Standard*. Reprinted in Blum, D. (2014), *The Best American Science and Nature Writing* (pp. 19–34). New York: Houghton Mifflin Harcourt.

Dyson, F. (2015). The collapse of the wave function. In: J. Brockman (Ed.), *This Idea Must Die* (p. 73). New York: HarperCollins.

Erdman, D. V. (Ed.) (1988). *The Complete Poetry and Prose of William Blake, Newly Revised Edition*. New York: Random House.

Feinberg, T. E. (2010). Neuropathologies of the self: a general theory. *Neuropsychoanalysis, 12*: 133–158.

Ferris, J. (2015). First impressions. *Scientific American, 33*(1): 24.

Freud, S. (1900a). *The Interpretation of Dreams (Part Two), S. E., 5*: 339–622. London: Hogarth.

Freud, S. (1912e). Recommendations to physicians practising psychoanalysis. *S. E., 7*: 109–120. London: Hogarth.

Freud, S. (1915e). The unconscious. *S. E., 14*: 166–204. London: Hogarth.

Freud, S. (1917d). A metapsychological supplement to the theory of dreams. *S. E., 14*: 217–235. London: Hogarth.

Freud, S. (1920g). *Beyond the Pleasure Principle. S. E., 18*: 7–64. London: Hogarth.

Freud, S. (1925h). Negation. *S. E., 19*: 235–243. London: Hogarth.

Freud, S. (1927e). Fetishism. *S. E., 21*: 147–158. London: Hogarth.

Freud, S. (1940a). *An Outline of Psychoanalysis. S. E., 23*: 14–207. London: Hogarth.

Friston, K. (2010). The free-energy principle: a unified brain theory? Nature Reviews. *Neuroscience, 11*: 127–138.

Friston, K. (2014). Consciousness and the Bayesian Brain==09—Sandler Conference, 2014. www.youtube.com/watch?v=HeQfO4byFhg (accessed 3 November 2015).

Giegerich, W., Miller, D. L., & Mogenson, G. (2005). 'Conflict/resolution,' 'opposites/creative union' versus dialectics, and the climb up the slippery mountain. In: *Dialectics and Analytical Psychology: The El Capitan Canyon Seminar*. New Orleans, LA: Spring Journal Books.

Green, A. (1992). Review of *Cogitations* by Wilfred R. Bion, edited with a Foreword by Francesca Bion. *International Journal of Psychoanalysis, 73*: 585–589.

Green, A. (1999). The work of the negative and hallucinatory activity (negative hallucination). In: *The Work of the Negative* (pp. 161–214). London: Free Association Books [reprinted in M. K. O'Neil & S. Akhtar (Eds.) (2011), *On Freud's "Negation"* (pp. 75–144). London: Karnac].

Greenblatt, S. (2011). *The Swerve: How the World Became Modern*. New York: W. W. Norton.

Gurevich, H. (2008). The language of absence. *International Journal of Psychoanalysis, 89*: 561–578.

Heidegger, M. (1996). *Being and Time: A Translation of* Sein und Zeit, J. Stambaugh (Trans.). New York: State University of New York Press.

Hinshelwood, R. D. (2008). Repression and splitting: towards a method of conceptual comparison. *International Journal of Psychoanalysis, 89*: 503–521.

Hobson, J. A. (1994). *The Chemistry of Conscious States: How the Brain Changes its Mind*. Boston, MA: Little, Brown.

Hollander, R., & Hollander, J. (Trans.) (2000). *The Inferno*. New York: Anchor Books.

Hut, P. (2014). Interview with Piet Hut, in Second Life format. (21 October) https://wiki.playasbeing.org/chronicles/the_chapter_31:_pema_pera_interview (accessed 28 October 2015).

Joseph, R. (1992). The limbic system: emotion, laterality, and unconscious mind. *Psychoanalytic Review, 79*: 405–456.

Jospiovic, Z., Dinstein, I., Weber, J., & Heeger, D. J. (2012). Influence of meditation on anti-correlated networks in the brain. *Frontiers in Human Neuroscience, 5*: 1–11.

Kaplan-Solms, K., & Solms, M. (2000). *Clinical Studies in Neuro-Psychoanalysis: Introduction to a Depth Neuropsychology*. London: Karnac.

Kaufman, J., Yang, B. Z., Douglas-Palumberi, H., Houshyar, S., Lipschitz, D., Krystal, J. H., & Gelernter, J. (2004). Social supports and serotonin transporter gene moderate depression in maltreated children. *Proceedings of the National Academy of Sciences, 101*(49): 17316–17321.

Laland, K., Uller, T., Feldman, F., Stereiny, K., Muller, G., Moczek, A., Joblonka, E., Odling-Smee, J., Wary, G., Hoekstra, H., Futuyma, D.,

Lenski, R., Makay, T., Schluter, D., & Strassmann, J. (2014). Does evolutionary theory need a rethink? *Nature*, *514*: 161–164. See *Nature* Comment, *514*(1721) at: www.nature.com/news/does–evolutionary–theory–need–a–rethink–1.16080 (accessed 28 October 2015).

Loewald, H. W. (1976). Perspectives on memory. In: *Papers on Psychoanalysis* (pp. 148–173). New Haven, CT: Yale University Press, 1980.

Mancia, M. (1981). On the beginning of mental life in the foetus. *International Journal of Psychoanalysis, 62*: 351–357.

Mancia, M. (1989). On the birth of the self. *Rivista di Psicoanalisi, 35*: 1052–1072.

Mancia, M. (2006). Implicit memory and early unrepressed unconscious: their role in the therapeutic process (how the neurosciences can contribute to psychoanalysis). *International Journal of Psychoanalysis, 87*: 83–103.

Matte-Blanco, I. (1988). *Thinking, Feeling, and Being: Clinical Reflections on the Fundamental Antinomy of Human Beings and World*. London: Tavistock/Routledge.

McGilchrist, I. (2009). *The Master and his Emissary*. New Haven, CT: Yale University Press.

Merleau-Ponty, M. (1945). *Phenomenology of Perception*, C. Smith (Trans.). New York: Routledge, 1995.

Milgram, S. (1974). *Obedience to Authority: An Experimental View*. New York: Harper Row.

Mills, J. (1996). Hegel on the unconscious abyss: implications for psychoanalysis. *The Owl and the Minerva, 28*: 59–75.

Mills, J. (2000). Hegel on projective identification: implications for Klein, Bion, and beyond. *Psychoanalytic Review, 87*: 841–874.

Mills, J. (2002). Deciphering the "genesis problem": on the dialectical origins of psychic reality. *Psychoanalytic Review, 89*: 763–809.

Nichols, W. (2014). *Blue Mind*. New York: Little, Brown.

O'Conner, D., Fukui, M., Pinsk, M., & Kastner, S. (2002). Attention modulates responses in the human lateral geniculate nucleus. *Nature Neuroscience, 5*: 1203–1209.

Ogden, T. H. (1992a). The dialectically constituted/decentered subject of psychoanalysis. I. The Freudian subject. *International Journal of Psychoanalysis, 73*: 517–526.

Ogden, T. H. (1992b). The dialectically constituted/decentered subject of psychoanalysis II. The contributions of Klein and Winnicott. *International Journal of Psychoanalysis, 73*: 613–626.

Ogden, T. H. (1994). *Subjects of Analysis*. Northvale, NJ: Jason Aronson.

Ogden, T. H. (1998). On the dialectical structure of experience: some clinical and theoretical implications. *Contemporary Psychoanalysis, 24*: 17–45.

Ogden, T. H. (2002). A new reading of the origins of object relations theory. *International Journal of Psychoanalysis, 83*: 767–782.

Ogden, T. H. (2004). An introduction to the reading of Bion. *International Journal of Psychoanalysis, 85*: 285–300.

Olinick, S. L. (1970). Negative therapeutic reaction. *Journal of the American Psychoanalytic Association, 18*: 655–672.

O'Neil, M. K., & Akhtar, S. (2011). *On Freud's "Negation"*. London: Karnac.

Pally, R. (1997). Memory: brain systems that link past, present and future. *International Journal of Psycho-Analysis, 78*: 1223–1234.

Pally, R. (1998). Emotional processing: the mind–body connection. *International Journal of Psychoanalysis, 79*: 349–362.

Pally, R. (2010). Frontline—the brain's shared circuits of interpersonal understanding: implications for psychoanalysis and psychodynamic psychotherapy. *Journal of the American Academy of Psychoanalysis, 38*: 381–411.

Panksepp, J. (2013). Toward an understanding of the constitution of consciousness through the laws of affect. *Neuropsychoanalysis, 15*: 62–65.

Plato (1965). *Timaeus and Critias*, D. Lee (Trans.). Harmondsworth: Penguin Classics, 1987.

Reis, B. E. (1999). Thomas Ogden's phenomenological turn. *Psychoanalytic Dialogues, 9*: 371–393.

Ricard, M., Lutz, A., & Davidson, R. J. (2014). Mind of the meditator. *Scientific American, 311*(5): 39–45.

Rosenfeld, H. (1987). *Impasse and Interpretation*. New York: Routledge.

Sacks, O. (2008). *Musicophilia: Tales of Music and the Brain* (revised and expanded). New York: Vintage Books.

Salas, C., & Turnbull, O. H. (2010). In self-defense: disruptions in the sense of self, lateralization, and primitive defenses. *Neuropsychoanalysis, 12*: 172–182.

Sandler, P. (2005). *The Language of Bion: A Dictionary of Concepts*. London: Karnac.

Sandler, P. (2015). Commentary on "Transformations in hallucinosis and the receptivity of the analyst" by Civitarese. *International Journal of Psychoanalysis, 96*: 1139–1157.

Schmidt, C. (2015). Mental health may depend on creatures in the gut. *Scientific American, 312*(3): S12–S15.

Schore, A. N. (Ed.) (1994). *Affect Regulation and the Origin of the Self*. Mahwah, NJ: Lawence Erlbaum.

Schore, A. N. (2002). Advances in neuropsychoanalysis, attachment theory, and trauma research: implications for self psychology. *Psychoanalytic Inquiry, 22*: 433–484.

Schore, A. N. (2011). The right brain implicit self lies at the core of psychoanalysis. *Psychoanalytic Dialogues, 21*: 75–100.

Schwab, K., Groh, T., Schwab, M., & Witte, H. (2009). Nonlinear analysis and modeling of cortical activation and deactivation patterns in the immature fetal electrocorticogram. *Chaos: An Interdisciplinary Journal of Nonlinear Science,* 2009; 19 (1): 015111 DOI: 10.1063/1.3100546 [reprinted in American Institute of Physics. Baby's first dreams: sleep cycles of the fetus. *Science Daily,* 14 April 2009].

Siegel, D. (2012). *The Developing Mind: How Relationships and the Brain Interact to Shape Who We Are* (2nd edn). New York: Guildford Press.

Simon, D., & Chabris, C. (1999). www.theinvisiblegorilla.com/videos.html (video, accessed 1 October 2015).

Singer, J. A., & Conway, M. A. (2011). Reconsidering therapeutic action: Loewald, cognitive neuroscience and the integration of memory's duality. *International Journal of Psychoanalysis, 92*: 1183–1207.

Smith, M. F. (Trans.) (1969). *Lucretius, On the Nature of Things.* London: Sphere Books [reprinted Indianapolis, IN: Hackett, 2001].

Solms, M. (1997). What is consciousness? *Journal of the American Psychoanalytic Association, 45*: 681–703.

Solms, M. (2013). The Conscious Id. *Neuropsychoanalysis, 15*: 5–19.

Solms, M., & Turnbull, O. (2002). *The Brain and the Inner World: An Introduction to the Neuroscience of Subjective Experience.* New York: Other Press.

Spillius, E. B., Milton, J., Garvey, P., Couve, C., & Steiner, D. (2011). *The New Dictionary of Kleinian Thought.* London: Routledge.

Steiner, G. (1978). *Martin Heidegger,* New York: Viking.

Trevarthen, C. (1996). Lateral asymmetries in infancy: implications for the development of the hemispheres. *Neuroscience and Biobehavioral Reviews, 20*(4): 571–586.

Tweedy, R. (2012). *The God of the Left Hemisphere: Blake, Bolte Taylor and the Myth of Creation.* London: Karnac.

Vermote, R. (2011). Rudi Vermote's response to David Taylor. *International Journal of Psychoanalysis, 92*: 1113–1116.

Weinhold, B. (2006). Epigenetics: the science of change. *Environmental Health Perspectives, 114*(3): A160–167.

Weston, D., & Gabbard, G. O. (2002). Developments in cognitive neuroscience: I. Conflict, compromise, and connectionism. *Journal of the American Psychoanalytic Association, 50*: 53–98.

Winnicott, D. W. (1949). Mind and its relation to the psyche–soma. In: *Collected Papers: Through Paediatrics to Psycho-analysis* (pp. 243–254). London: Hogarth, 1958.

Winnicott, D. W. (1953). Transitional objects and transitional phenomena —a study of the first not-me possession. *International Journal of Psychoanalysis, 34*: 89–97.

Winnicott, D. W. (1960). The theory of the parent–infant relationship. *International Journal of Psychoanalysis, 41*: 585–595.

Zimbardo, P. (2007). *The Lucifer Effect: Understanding How Good People Turn Evil.* New York: Random House.

INDEX